DNA Microarrays

The Practical Approach Series

SERIES EDITOR

B. D. HAMES
Department of Biochemistry and Molecular Biology
University of Leeds, Leeds LS2 9JT, UK

See also the Practical Approach web site at **http://www.oup.co.uk/PAS**
★ **indicates new and forthcoming titles**

Affinity Chromatography
Affinity Separations
Anaerobic Microbiology
Animal Cell Culture
  (2nd edition)
Animal Virus Pathogenesis
Antibodies I and II
Antibody Engineering
★ Antisense Technology
Applied Microbial Physiology
Basic Cell Culture
Behavioural Neuroscience
Bioenergetics
Biological Data Analysis
Biomechanics—Materials
Biomechanics—Structures and
  Systems
Biosensors
Carbohydrate Analysis
  (2nd edition)
Cell–Cell Interactions
The Cell Cycle
Cell Growth and Apoptosis
★ Cell Separation

Cellular Calcium
Cellular Interactions in
  Development
Cellular Neurobiology
★ Chromatin
★ Chromosome Structural
  Analysis
Clinical Immunology
Complement
★ Crystallization of Nucleic
  Acids and Proteins
  (2nd edition)
Cytokines (2nd edition)
The Cytoskeleton
Diagnostic Molecular
  Pathology I and II
DNA and Protein Sequence
  Analysis
DNA Cloning 1: Core
  Techniques (2nd edition)
DNA Cloning 2: Expression
  Systems (2nd edition)
DNA Cloning 3: Complex
  Genomes (2nd edition)
DNA Cloning 4: Mammalian
  Systems (2nd edition)

DNA Microarrays

A Practical Approach

Edited by

MARK SCHENA

Department of Biochemistry, Beckman Center, Stanford University
Medical Center, Stanford, USA

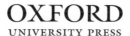

OXFORD
UNIVERSITY PRESS

OXFORD

UNIVERSITY PRESS

Great Clarendon Street, Oxford OX2 6DP

Oxford University Press is a department of the University of Oxford
and furthers the University's aim of excellence in research, scholarship,
and education by publishing worldwide in

Oxford New York

Athens Auckland Bangkok Bogotá Buenos Aires Calcutta
Cape Town Chennai Dar es Salaam Delhi Florence Hong Kong Istanbul
Karachi Kuala Lumpur Madrid Melbourne Mexico City Mumbai
Nairobi Paris São Paulo Singapore Taipei Tokyo Toronto Warsaw

and associated companies in Berlin Ibadan

Oxford is a registered trade mark of Oxford University Press

Published in the United States
by Oxford University Press Inc., New York

© Oxford University Press 1999
Reprinted 2000 (three times)

Users of books in the Practical Approach Series are advised that prudent
laboratory safety procedures should be followed at all times. Oxford
University Press makes no representation, express or implied, in respect of
the accuracy of the material set forth in books in this series and cannot
accept any legal responsibility or liability for any errors or omissions
that may be made.

A catalogue record for this book is available from the British Library

Library of Congress Cataloging in Publication Data
DNA microarrays : a practical approach / edited by Mark Schena.
(Practical approach series ; 205)
Includes bibliographical references.
1. DNA microarrays.   I. Schena, Mark.   II. Series.
QP624.5.D726D63   572.8'65—dc21   99–13842

ISBN 0-19-963777-6 (Hbk)
         0-19-963776-8 (Pbk)

Printed in Great Britain by Information Press, Ltd,
Eynsham, Oxon.

Preface

I was 14 years old in the summer of 1977, and it was then that a neighbour first told me about the Stanford Biochemistry Department. Stanford chemistry majors were required to take a class outside their field of immediate study and he opted for a course in biochemistry. Because I had already decided to pursue a career in biochemistry—indeed well before I knew what biochemistry was—it seemed reasonable to ask him about the experience. He said flatly that he enjoyed the course...except for all the biochemistry. And so it was. I was determined to seek out biochemistry and to cross paths with the lauded department that housed the likes of Baldwin, Berg, Hogness, Kaiser, Kornberg, and Lehman.

Enter a spring day in Berkeley in 1983 and a nervous Assistant Professor who had recently completed post-doctoral work at Stanford. Without asking, he volunteered that he had worked for Ron Davis and described him as the 'world's smartest biochemist'. I double checked with Koshland and he confirmed Ron's growing reputation as an enigmatic and brilliant investigator. Later that day and still under the legal drinking age, I had a beer (illegally) and pondered how it was that I would eventually manage to work for Davis.

The UCSF shunt proved unexpectedly prosperous, hitting pay dirt with Yamamoto at an early stage of graduate training. It was in San Francisco, under Yamamoto's stern direction, that I learned how to do science. Marinated in a tonic of Alberts, Bishop, Herskowitz, Pruisner, Varmus, and others, it was difficult *not* to be successful at UCSF.

It was late in 1993 that the daunting complexity of plant transcript factor function led us to some serious pondering and triggered the insane idea that gene expression might best be studied with DNA chips. The notion drew audible laughter from a crowd of 500 in Holland during the summer of 1994. Charging ahead with support from Fodor, Shalon, and Brown, we managed to move the project from infancy to publication in October of 1995.

At present, the microarray field is growing rapidly, fueled internationally by contributors from both academia and industry. The stage is set for a fundamental transformation of biology from a gene science into a genome science. Drawing steadily on expertise from chemistry, engineering, and physics, biochip assays are fast becoming sophisticated and affordable. It is a great privilege to edit a timely book on this subject. Oxford University Press and each of the talented contributors have me wondering, as I have so many times in the past, how it is that I always seem to get much more from science than I deserve.

Stanford   M. S.
April 1999

Contents

3. Representational differences analysis and microarray hybridization for efficient cloning and screening of differentially expressed genes   43

Stanley F. Nelson and Christopher T. Denny

Contents

4. Use of oligonucleotide arrays in enzymatic assays: assay optimization   61

Stephen Case-Green, Clare Pritchard, and Edwin M. Southern

5. Antisense oligonucleotide scanning arrays   77

John K. Elder, Martin Johnson, Natalie Milner, Kalim U. Mir, Muhammad Sohail, and Edwin M. Southern

Contents

8. Expression data and the bioinformatics challenges

Joel Lloyd Bellenson

9. Active microelectronic arrays for DNA hybridization analysis

Michael J. Heller, Eugene Tu, Anita Holmsen, Ronald G. Sosnowski, and James O'Connell

10. Gene chips and microarrays: applications in disease profiles, drug target discovery, drug action and toxicity

Renu A. Heller, John Allard, Fengrong Zuo, Christopher Lock, Stacy Wilson, Paul Klonowski, Hans Gmuender, Harold Van Wart, and Robert Booth

Contents

Contributors

JOHN ALLARD
Inflammatory Diseases Unit, Roche Bioscience, 3401 Hillview Avenue, Palo Alto, CA 94304, USA.

JOEL LLOYD BELLENSON
Pangea Systems Inc., 1999 Harrison Street, Suite 1100, Oakland, CA 94612, USA.

ANTON BITTNER
R. W. Johnson Pharmaceutical Research Institute, 3535 General Atomics Court, Suite 100, San Diego, CA 92121, USA.

ROBERT BOOTH
Inflammatory Diseases Unit, Roche Bioscience, 3401 Hillview Avenue, Palo Alto, CA 94304, USA.

STEPHEN CASE-GREEN
Department of Biochemistry, University of Oxford, South Parks Road, Oxford OX1 3QU, UK.

JIM R. CHAMBERS
R. W. Johnson Pharmaceutical Research Institute, 3535 General Atomics Court, Suite 100, San Diego, CA 92121, USA.

RONALD W. DAVIS
Department of Biochemistry, Beckman Center, Stanford University Medical Center, Stanford, CA 94305-5307, USA.

CHRISTOPHER T. DENNY
University of California, Los Angeles, UCLA Medical Center, 710 Westwood Plaza, Los Angeles, CA 90095-1769, USA.

JOHN K. ELDER
Department of Biochemistry, University of Oxford, South Parks Road, Oxford OX1 3QU, UK.

MARK G. ERLANDER
R. W. Johnson Pharmaceutical Research Institute, 3535 General Atomics Court, Suite 100, San Diego, CA 92121, USA.

RONALD C. GAMBLE
Gamble & Associates Ltd., LLC 2038 Foothill Blvd., Pasadena, CA 91107, USA.

HANS GMUENDER
PRPI, F. Hoffmann-La Roche Ltd., Basel, CH-4070, Switzerland.

Contributors

HONGQING GUO
R. W. Johnson Pharmaceutical Research Institute, 3535 General Atomics Court, Suite 100, San Diego, CA 92121, USA.

MICHAEL J. HELLER
Nanogen, 10398 Pacific Center Court, San Diego, CA 92121, USA.

RENU A. HELLER
Inflammatory Diseases Unit, Roche Bioscience, 3401 Hillview Avenue, Palo Alto, CA 94304, USA.

ANITA HOLMSEN
Nanogen, 10398 Pacific Center Court, San Diego, CA 92121, USA.

MICHAEL R. JACKSON
R. W. Johnson Pharmaceutical Research Institute, 3535 General Atomics Court, Suite 100, San Diego, CA 92121, USA.

MARTIN JOHNSON
Department of Biochemistry, University of Oxford, South Parks Road, Oxford OX1 3QU, UK.

K. C. JOY
R. W. Johnson Pharmaceutical Research Institute, 3535 General Atomics Court, Suite 100, San Diego, CA 92121, USA.

PAUL KLONOWSKI
Inflammatory Diseases Unit, Roche Bioscience, 3401 Hillview Avenue, Palo Alto, CA 94304, USA.

CHRISTOPHER LOCK
Department of Neurology and Neurological Sciences, Stanford University School of Medicine, Stanford, CA 94305, USA.

LIN LUO
R. W. Johnson Pharmaceutical Research Institute, 3535 General Atomics Court, Suite 100, San Diego, CA 92121, USA.

NATALIE MILNER
Department of Biochemistry, University of Oxford, South Parks Road, Oxford OX1 3QU, UK.

KALIM U. MIR
Department of Biochemistry, University of Oxford, South Parks Road, Oxford OX1 3QU, UK.

STANLEY F. NELSON
University of California, Los Angeles, UCLA Medical Center, 710 Westwood Plaza, Los Angeles, CA 90095-1769, USA.

Contributors

JAMES O'CONNELL
Nanogen, 10398 Pacific Center Court, San Diego, CA 92121, USA.

CLARE PRITCHARD
Department of Biochemistry, University of Oxford, South Parks Road, Oxford OX1 3QU, UK.

RANELLE C. SALUNGA
R. W. Johnson Pharmaceutical Research Institute, 3535 General Atomics Court, Suite 100, San Diego, CA 92121, USA.

MARK SCHENA
Department of Biochemistry, Beckman Center, Stanford University Medical Center, Stanford, CA 94305-5307, USA.

MACK J. SCHERMER
Life Science Products Group, General Scanning, Inc., 500 Arsenal Street, Watertown, MA 02472, USA.

MUHAMMAD SOHAIL
Department of Biochemistry, University of Oxford, South Parks Road, Oxford OX1 3QU, UK.

RONALD G. SOSNOWSKI
Nanogen, 10398 Pacific Center Court, San Diego, CA 92121, USA.

EDWIN M. SOUTHERN
Department of Biochemistry, University of Oxford, South Parks Road, Oxford OX1 3QU, UK.

THOMAS P. THERIAULT
Incyte Pharmaceuticals, Inc., Microarray Systems, 6519 Dumbarton Circle, Fremont, CA 94555, USA.

EUGENE TU
Nanogen, 10398 Pacific Center Court, San Diego, CA 92121, USA.

HAROLD VAN WART
Inflammatory Diseases Unit, Roche Bioscience, 3401 Hillview Avenue, Palo Alto, CA 94304, USA.

JACKSON S. WAN
R. W. Johnson Pharmaceutical Research Institute, 3535 General Atomics Court, Suite 100, San Diego, CA 92121, USA.

STACY WILSON
Inflammatory Diseases Unit, Roche Bioscience, 3401 Hillview Avenue, Palo Alto, CA 94304, USA.

Contributors

SCOTT C. WINDER
Incyte Pharmaceuticals, Inc., Microarray Systems, 6519 Dumbarton Circle, Fremont, CA 94555, USA.

FENGRONG ZUO
Inflammatory Diseases Unit, Roche Bioscience, 3401 Hillview Avenue, Palo Alto, CA 94304, USA.

Abbreviations

APD	avalanche photodiodes
BSA	bovine serum albumin
CCD	charge-coupled device
DEPC	diethyl pyrocarbonate
EST	expressed sequence tag
FITC	fluorescein isothiocyanate
LCM	laser capture microdissection
NA	numerical aperture
PCR	polymerase chain reaction
PMT	photomultiplier tube
PR	photoresist
RDA	representational difference analysis
RT	room temperature
SNP	single nucleotide polymorphism
SSH	subtractive suppressive hybridization
STR	short tandem repeat

1

Genes, genomes, and chips

MARK SCHENA and RONALD W. DAVIS

1. Introduction

This chapter provides an overview of the microarray or biochip field, describing biological framework, historical perspective, applications, and future trends. Microarray assays are summarized and compared to traditional approaches. Methodological underpinnings of biochips are emphasized.

2. Information content of genomes

2.1 DNA

The information content of the genome is carried hereditarily as deoxyribonucleic acid (DNA). The size and composition of a given genomic sequence determines the form and function of the resultant organism. In general, genomic complexity is proportional to the complexity of the organism. Relatively simple organisms such as bacteria have genomes in the 1–5 million base (megabase) range while mammalian genomes including human are approximately 3000 megabases; genomes from organisms of intermediate complexity such as worms and insects are typically 100–200 megabases.

The genome is generally divided into distinct segments known as chromosomes. The bacterium *Escherichia coli* (*E. coli*) contains a single circular chromosome, whereas the yeast *Saccharomyces cerevisiae* contains 16 linear chromosomes. The human genome consists of 23 autosomes and one sex chromosome, such that the 24 human chromosomes contain all of the 3000 megabases of the human genome.

Genomic DNA exists as a double-stranded polymer containing four DNA bases (A, G, C, and T) tethered to a sugar-phosphate backbone (*Table 1*). The order of the bases along the DNA is known as the primary sequence of the DNA. The main goal of the Human Genome Project is to determine the primary sequence of all three billion bases comprising the 24 chromosomes of the human genome. Genome sequencing, also known as structural genomics, provides the sequence information for the biochip industry (see Sections 3–6).

The two strands of genomic DNA are held together by hydrogen bonding

Table 1. Information content of genomes

Information	DNA	RNA	Protein
Hereditary blueprint	Complete	Partial	Partial
Genomic representation[a]	100%	3%	3%
Type	Coding and non-coding	Coding only	Coding only
Form	Double-stranded	Single-stranded	Folded
Composition	Nucleic acid	Nucleic acid	Amino acid
Hybridization	Yes	Yes	No
Bases	A, G, C, T	A, G, C, U	Not applicable
Total building blocks	4	4	20
Ploidy effect[b]	Yes	Yes	Yes
Transcriptional effect[b]	No	Yes	Yes
Translational effect[b]	No	No	Yes
Biochemical modifications	Methylation	Polyadenylation, capping	Phosphorylation, acylation
Microarray assays	Yes	Yes	No[c]

[a] For human.
[b] Excludes secondary effects.
[c] Published.

interactions between complementary bases on each strand. The chemical structure of the bases is such that A interacts with T (and not with any of the other bases) and G interacts with C (and not with any of the other bases). The inherent double-stranded conformation of DNA and the precision of the base pairing interactions can be exploited in a process known as hybridization (1). Hybridization is the process by which two complementary, single-stranded nucleic acid chains form a stable double helix. Hybridization reactions can occur between two complementary molecules in solution or between a molecule in solution and a complementary molecule immobilized on a solid support. Because DNA chip assays utilize hybridization reactions between single-stranded fluorescent molecules and single-stranded sequences on the chip surface, hybridization is the biochemical process on which the entire DNA microarray industry is based (see Section 3).

The genome of an organism contains both protein coding and non-coding regions (*Table 1*) and thus includes exons and introns, promoter and gene regulatory regions, origins of replication, telomeres, and non-functional intergenic DNA. Genome analysis can provide a quantitative measure of gene copy number and chromosome number or ploidy, as well as the presence of single base differences in the primary sequence of the DNA. Single base changes that are inherited are generally referred to as polymorphisms, whereas those that are acquired during the life of an organism are commonly known as mutations. In one view, genome analysis provides a detailed picture of the *genetic potential* of an organism by delineating the precise nucleotide sequence of all the genes and gene regulatory regions. Genomic analysis at the DNA level does

2

not, however, provide a measure of gene expression which is the process by which RNA and protein copies of the coding sequences are synthesized (see Sections 2.2 and 2.3).

All of the cells from a given organism are generally assumed to contain identical genomes, while genomes from different individuals of the same species are typically ~ 99.9% identical. The 0.1% polymorphism rate among individuals (2) is significant in that approximately three million polymorphisms (three billion bases × 0.1%) are expected to be found upon complete sequencing of any two human genomes. If single base changes occur in protein coding segments, polymorphisms can alter the protein sequence and therefore change the biochemical activity of the gene products. Assuming that the human genome contains ~ 3% coding sequences and that ~ 1% of the polymorphisms alter protein function, each human in the population is expected to contain approximately 900 gene products with altered activity. Because the function of the gene products underlies all aspects of human health, polymorphism detection is a central aspect of functional genomics.

2.2 RNA

The DNA genome consists of discrete functional regions known as genes. Genomes of simple organisms such as bacteria contain 1000–3000 genes (3), whereas the human genome is estimated to contain 50 000–100 000 genes (4). Multicellular organisms including yeast, flies, and worms contain 5000–25 000 genes (5).

Gene expression is the process by which messenger RNA (mRNA) and eventually protein is synthesized from the DNA template of each gene. mRNA is a single-stranded molecule consisting of four DNA bases tethered to a sugar-phosphate backbone (*Table 1*). The portion of each gene that is represented as mRNA is known as the coding sequence for that gene. Approximately 3% of the human genome is represented as coding sequence (*Table 1*).

Because mRNA is an exact copy of the DNA coding regions, mRNA analysis can be used to identify polymorphisms in coding regions of DNA; more importantly, genomic analysis at the mRNA level can be used as a measure of gene expression. Expression levels for each gene are dictated physiologically by a combination of genetic and environmental factors. The genetic factors that determine gene expression activity include the precise DNA sequence of gene regulatory regions such as promoters, enhancers, and splice sites. Polymorphisms in the DNA are thus expected to contribute some of the differences in gene expression among individuals of the same species. Expression levels are also affected by a large number of environmental factors, including temperature, stress, light, and other signals, that lead to changes in the levels of hormones and other signalling substances. For this reason, RNA analysis provides information not only about the genetic potential of an organism, but also about dynamic changes in *functional state*.

3

Each human cell can be viewed as a functional unit containing 50 000–100 000 gene variables, whose expression level determines the functional state of the cell (6). For most genes, steady state mRNA levels approximate protein levels and thus quantitative expression monitoring at the mRNA level provides important clues as to function. Specific changes in mRNA have been documented as a function of heat shock, drug treatment, and metabolic and disease states (7). The hypothesis that many or all human diseases may be accompanied by specific changes in gene expression (8) has generated much commercial interest in gene expression monitoring at the whole genome level. The ease of obtaining fluorescent probes from mRNA (*Protocol 1*) and the ease by which these probes can be analysed by hybridization-based assays (9–17), has catapulted mRNA monitoring into a limelight activity in functional genomics.

Protocol 1. Fluorescent probe preparation from messenger RNA

Equipment and reagents

- StrataScript RT–PCR kit (Stratagene)
- Oligo(dT) 21-mer (treated with 0.1% DEPC to inactivate ribonucleases)
- 100 mM dATP, dCTP, dGTP, dTTP (Pharmacia)
- 1 mM Cy3-dCTP (Amersham)
- 1 mM Cy5-dCTP (Amersham)
- 1 mM fluorescein-12-dCTP (DuPont)
- SuperScript II RNase H, reverse transcriptase (Gibco BRL)

Method

1. In an Eppendorf tube, mix 5 μl total mRNA (1 μg/μl),[a] 1 μl control mRNA cocktail (0.5 ng/μl),[b] 4 μl oligo(dT) 21-mer (1 μg/μl), and 17 μl H$_2$O (DEPC treated) for a total volume of 27 μl.

2. Denature mRNA by heating for 3 min at 65°C.

3. Anneal oligo(dT) to mRNA by incubating for 10 min at 25°C.

4. Add 10 μl 5 × first strand buffer, 5 μl 10 × DTT (0.1 M), 1.5 μl RNase block (20 U/μl), 1 μl cocktail of dATP, dGTP, dTTP (25 mM each), 2 μl dCTP (1 mM), 2 μl Cy3-dCTP (1 mM),[c] 1.5 μl SuperScript II reverse transcriptase (200 U/μl) for a total reaction volume of 50 μl.

5. Reverse transcribe for 2 h at 37°C.

6. Add 5 μl 2.5 M sodium acetate and 110 μl 100% ethanol at 25°C.[d]

7. Centrifuge for 15 min at 25°C in a microcentrifuge to pellet cDNA: mRNA hybrids.[e]

8. Remove and discard supernatant and carefully wash pellet with 0.5 ml 80% ethanol.[f]

9. Dry pellet in a SpeedVac and resuspend in 10 μl 1 × TE pH 8.[g,h]

10. Boil sample for 3 min to denature cDNA:mRNA hybrids. Chill on ice immediately.

11. Add 2.5 μl 1 M NaOH and incubate for 10 min at 37 °C to degrade the mRNA.

12. Neutralize the cDNA mixture by adding 2.5 μl 1 M Tris–HCl pH 6.8 and 2 μl 1 M HCl.

13. Add 1.7 μl 2.5 M sodium acetate and 37 μl 100% ethanol.

14. Centrifuge for 15 min at full speed in a microcentrifuge to pellet the cDNA.[e]

15. Remove and discard supernatant and wash pellet with 0.5 ml 80% ethanol.[f]

16. Dry pellet in a SpeedVac and resuspend in 6.5 μl H$_2$O.

17. Add 2.5 μl 20 × SSC and 1 μl 2% SDS.

18. Heat at 65 °C for 0.5 min to dissolve probe mixture.

19. Centrifuge for 2 min in a microcentrifuge at high speed to pellet trace debris.[i]

20. Transfer supernatant to a new tube (probe concentration ∼ 0.5 μg/μl in 5 × SSC and 0.2% SDS).

[a] Total mRNA purified from total RNA using Oligotex-dT.
[b] Cocktail contains a dilution series of *Arabidopsis* mRNAs transcribed *in vitro*.
[c] To label mRNA with other fluors, substitute Fl12- or Cy5-dCTP in the reaction.
[d] Chilling or use of > 2 vol. ethanol results in precipitation of free label.
[e] Pellet product on one side of the tube, then remove supernatant from the *other side*.
[f] To prevent loss of pellet, centrifuge for 1 min before removing 80% ethanol.
[g] Product often smears up the *side* of the tube. Resuspend thoroughly!
[h] Resuspend the fluorescein, Cy3, or Cy5 labelled products in 10 μl total volume.
[i] Tiny particles interfere with hybridization, which is carried out under a coverslip.

2.3 Protein

The second step in gene expression is the synthesis of protein from mRNA. A unique protein is encoded by each mRNA, such that every three nucleotides of mRNA encodes one amino acid of the polypeptide chain. A 999 nucleotide mRNA will thus form a 333 amino acid protein, with the linear order of the nucleotides represented as a linear sequence of amino acids. Once synthesized, the protein assumes a unique three-dimensional conformation that is determined largely by the primary amino acid sequence. Once folded, proteins impart the functional instructions of the genome by performing a wide range of biochemical activities including roles in gene regulation, metabolism, cell structure, and DNA replication.

Individuals in a population are expected to have differences in protein activity due to polymorphisms which either alter the primary amino acid sequence of the proteins or perturb steady state protein levels by altering gene expression. Similar to mRNA levels, protein levels can also change in response to changes in the environment; moreover, protein levels are also subject to translational and post-translational control which do not effect mRNA levels directly (*Table 1*). Understanding protein activity thus requires information beyond what is obtained by studying DNA or RNA (*Table 1*).

One important level of post-translation control involves the covalent modification of proteins, whereby small molecular weight substituents such as phosphates, acyl groups, and the like are attached enzymatically to the amino acid side chains (*Table 1*). Covalent modification can alter the biochemical activity of proteins and thus the functional state of the cell. Because proteins ultimately impart the instructions of the genome, assessing protein activity is central to understanding genomic function. Unlike DNA and RNA, however, the protein activity cannot be measured by hybridization analysis (*Table 1*). High throughput, parallel protein analysis with microarrays poses a formidable technical challenge that so far has proven elusive (see Section 4).

3. Microarray assays

3.1 Substrate

Traditional hybridization assays developed in the 1970s utilize flexible membranes such as nitrocellulose and nylon, radioactivity, and autoradiography (18, 19). By contrast, microarray or biochip assays (*Figure 1*) utilize solid surfaces such as glass with fluorescent labelling and detection (9, 20). Compared to the macroscopic format of filter-based assays, the miniaturized biochip format represents a fundamental revolution in biological analysis (*Table 2*).

One advantage of the chip formats is that the solid surface is non-porous and thus enables the deposition small amounts of biochemical material in a precisely defined location (see Section 3.2). Porous substrates such as nylon

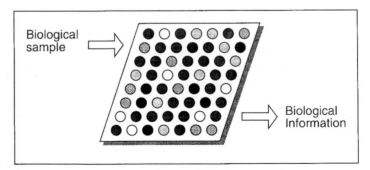

Figure 1. Concept of microarray assays. A biological sample is labelled with a fluorescent tag and reacted with a molecular microarray on a solid support. The location and extent of binding of the molecules on the microarray provide a quantitative measure of the identity and amount of gene or gene product present in the sample. Biological information such as gene expression and polymorphism data at the genomic level can be used to accelerate drug discovery, diagnostics, pharmacogenomics, and other important areas of biomedical research.

Table 2. Filter and microarray assays

Criterion	Filter	Microarray
Surface	Porous	Non-porous
Substrate	Non-uniform	Uniform
Conformation	Flexible	Solid
Format	Semi-parallel	Parallel
Compatible with miniaturization	No	Yes
Compatible with photolithograpy	No	Yes
Compatible with piezoelectric	No	Yes
Compatible with microspotting	No	Yes
Amenable to automated production	No	Yes
Compatible with fluorescence	No	Yes
Amenable to confocal scanning	No	Yes
Amenable to sample multiplexing	No	Yes
Sample concentration	Low	High
Hybridization kinetics	Slow	Fast
Reagent volumes	Large	Small
Data acquisition	Slow	Fast

and nitrocellulose allow diffusion of applied materials and are not amenable to microarray preparation. A non-porous substrate also prevents the absorption of reagents and sample into the substrate matrix, allowing the rapid removal of organic and fluorescent compounds during biochip fabrication and use (see Section 3.2). A non-porous surface permits the use of small sample volumes (*Table 2*), enabling high sample concentrations and rapid hybridization kinetics (see Section 3.3). A solid substrate also provides a uniform attachment surface which increases the quality of the array elements (*Table 2*). The inherent flatness of the microarray format permits true parallelism (*Figure 1*), which is lacking in all filter-based assays (*Table 2*). Parallel analysis provides a significant increase in the accuracy of the assay data (see Section 3.4).

3.2 Microarray fabrication

The biochip format is compatible with many advanced fabrication technologies and is thus amenable to automated manufacture (21). The three primary technologies used presently in microarray manufacture include photolithography, ink-jetting, mechanical microspotting, and derivatives thereof (*Table 3*). Each technology has specific advantages and disadvantages in biochip fabrication (*Table 3*), though none of these technologies is compatible with the non-porous substrates used in traditional hybridization assays.

The photolithograpy approach relies on the use of semiconductor technologies in a biochip setting (*Table 3*). Photomasks direct spatially defined, solid phase DNA synthesis through the use of light which serves to activate modified phosphoramidite versions of the four DNA bases for DNA synthesis (22). Each coupling step results in the addition of a single base to growing chains at

7

Table 3. Microarray fabrication technologies

Criterion	Photolithography	Piezoelectric	Microspotting
Combinatorial synthesis	Yes	Yes	No
Ink-jetting	No	Yes	No
Surface printing	No	No	Yes
Masks needed	Yes	No	No
Sample tracking	No	No	Yes
Density (cm^{-2})	244000	10000	6500
Length restriction	~ 25 nt	None	None
Array elements	Oligos only	Oligos and cDNAs	Oligos and cDNAs
Prototyping cost	High	Moderate	Low
Applications	Gene expression, mutation detection	Gene expression, mutation detection	Gene expression, mutation detection
Commercial vendors	Affymetrix	Biodot,[a] Cartesian,[a] Incyte, Packard Instruments, Protogene, Rosetta,	Cartesian, Genetix, Genometrix, Gene Machines,Genetic Microsystems, Hyseq, Molecular Dynamics, Norgren Systems, Synteni, TeleChem

[a] Non-piezoelectric 'ink-jetting' technology.

thousands of defined locations (22). The piezoelectric technologies utilize versions of 'ink-jet' printing to dispense sub-nanolitre volumes of reagents to defined locations (*Table 3*). Electricity is used to deliver DNA bases, cDNAs, and other molecules via tiny delivery jets onto a solid surface (23). An XYZ motion control system directs the location of the jets during this non-contact printing process (23). The microspotting technologies rely on direct surface contact for microarray fabrication (*Table 3*). A printhead containing micro-spotting pins (*Figure 2*), capillaries, or tweezers allows transfer of pre-made substances from reagent trays onto solid surfaces (9, 20, 24, 25). An XYZ motion control system directs the preparation of microarrays of oligonu-cleotides (*Figure 3*), cDNAs, and other biomolecules (9, 20, 24, 25). Detailed descriptions of each of the technologies is provided in subsequent chapters (see Chapters 2–10).

All three technologies permit the manufacture of microarrays for mutation detection and gene expression applications, two main applications of biochips in functional genomics (25). The three technologies each enable sufficient density (*Table 3*) to provide single chips that represent the entire human genome. The variable requirements of throughput, density, cost, quality, flexi-bility, and other criteria dictate the use of one of the three technologies in a given setting (25). The flurry of commercial activity in microarray manu-facturing suggests that all three technologies will be used in the foreseeable

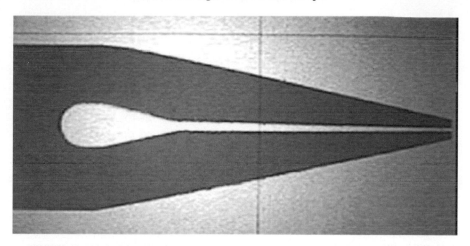

Figure 2. Bubble pin technology. Shown is the point of a 'bubble' microspotting pin (TeleChem) with an uptake channel fabricated into stainless steel. Liquid sample completely fills the uptake chamber, which is designed to hold a defined volume from 0.1–2 µl. Direct contact between the liquid and a solid surface deposits a drop of sample from the reservoir. The width of the point can be customized to deliver spots from 50–300 µm in diameter. The point shown here is 75 µm wide, which produces 100 µm features after sample spreading (see *Figure 3*).

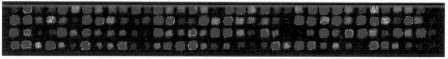

Figure 3. Microarray prepared by mechanical microspotting. Oligonucleotide microarray prepared with a microspotting pin (*Figure 2*) at 125 µm centre-to-centre spacing. Oligonucleotide concentrations equivalent to a range of 10 000–0.1 fluor/µm². Fluorescent scan obtained with the ScanArray 3000 (General Scanning) at 75% PMT and 70% laser power on the Cy3 channel. Data represented in a pseudocolour palette.

future (*Table 3*). In addition, advanced biosensor technologies also enable microarray experimentation (26). A description of one such platform is provided in Chapter 9.

3.3 Biochemical reactions

The biochemical reaction is the process whereby a sample of DNA or RNA isolated from a biological source is reacted with a biochip to yield an informative array of bound material (6). The inherent low level of intrinsic fluorescence of glass and other biochip substrates allows the use of fluorescent labelling and detection schemes in biochemical reactions involving microarrays (6, 8–17, 20, 25). The use of fluorescent labels, instead of radioisotopes which are used in traditional filter-based assays, provides a quantum leap in terms of speed, data quality, and user safety (6, 8–17, 20, 25).

Fluorescent labelling and detection exploits the availability of fluorescent versions of the DNA bases that absorb and emit light at distinct and separable wavelengths (27). Multicolour fluorescence in microarray assays permits the simultaneous analysis or multiplexing of two or more biological samples in a single assay (*Table 2*). Multiplexing can greatly increase the accuracy of results in both gene expression and mutation detection applications, by eliminating artefacts arising from chip-to-chip variation (8–10, 12–15, 28). Fluorescence-based assays also make it possible to exploit advanced data acquisition technologies (*Table 2*), including confocal scanning and imaging with charge-coupled device (CCD) cameras (Section 3.4).

Biochemical reactions in microarray assays benefit tremendously from the non-porous surfaces used in the chip approaches. Glass substrates permit the use of much smaller reaction volumes (5–200 μl) than are used in traditional filter assays (5–50 ml). Small reaction volumes reduce reagent consumption and cost, and increase the concentration of the nucleic acid reactants in microarray assays (0.1–1 μM) by as much as 100 000-fold compared to conventional assays (0.4–4 pM). Concentrated reactants accelerate hybridization kinetics, which reduces the length of time needed to obtain a strong fluorescent signal (*Table 2*). Glass substrates allow the use of coverslips sealed in reaction chambers for the hybridization reactions (*Protocol 2*).

Protocol 2. Hybridization reactions for expression monitoring

Equipment and reagents
- 22 mm cover glasses (Corning)
- Hybridization cassettes (TeleChem)
- Wash station (TeleChem)
- ScanArray 3000 (General Scanning)

Method

1. Place the 1″ × 3″ array in a hybridization chamber.[a]

2. Add 3 μl 0.1% SDS to the bottom of the array for humidification.[b]

3. Aliquot 5 μl fluorescent probe (*Protocol 1*) onto the 22 mm cover glass.

4. Carefully place the cover glass with probe over the array using forceps.[c,d]

5. Seal the hybridization cassette with the clear lid and tighten the four cassette screws.[a]

6. Submerge the hybridization cassette in a water-bath set at 62 °C.

7. Hybridize for 6 h at 62 °C.

8. Following hybridization, remove the array from the hybridization chamber.

9. Place the array *immediately* into the wash station.[e]

---

10. Wash the array with 400 ml 1 × SSC and 0.1% SDS for 5 min at room temperature.[f]

11. Transfer the array to a second beaker containing 400 ml 0.1 × SSC and 0.1% SDS.

12. Wash the array by gentle buffer agitation for 5 min at room temperature.

13. Rinse the array briefly in a third beaker containing 0.1 × SSC to remove the SDS.

14. Allow the arrays to air dry.[g]

15. Scan for fluorescence emission using the ScanArray 3000.

[a] Purchased from TeleChem.
[b] Aliquot the 0.1% SDS into the slot of the cassette.
[c] Coverslips must be dust- and particle-free to allow even seating on the array.
[d] Air bubbles trapped under the coverslip exit after several minutes at 62 °C.
[e] Use the TeleChem wash station.
[f] Buffer agitation accomplished by placing the beaker on a stir plate.
[g] Cy3 or Cy5 arrays are scanned dry.

3.4 Detection and data analysis

Once the fluorescent sample is reacted with the microarray, the unbound material is washed away and the sample bound to each element on the chip is visualized by fluorescence detection. Confocal scanning devices (6, 8–17, 20–22, 25, 28) and CCD cameras (6) have both been used successfully for microarray detection.

The most common configuration of a confocal scanner utilizes laser excitation of a small region of the glass substrate ($\sim 100~\mu m^2$), such that the entire image is gathered by moving the substrate or the confocal lens (or both) across the substrate in two dimensions. Light emitted from the fluorescent sample at each location is separated from unwanted light using a series of mirrors, filter, and lenses, and the light is converted to an electrical signal with a photomultiplier tube (PMT) or an equivalent detector. The speed of data gathering with a confocal scanner (1–5 min) is orders of magnitude faster than autoradiography with radioactive filters used in conventional experiments (one to ten days). Rapid fluorescent detection technology is a revolutionary aspect of microarray technology.

Fluorescent imaging with a CCD camera uses many of the same principles as a confocal scanner, though key details are different in both excitation and detection technology. One difference is that CCD-based imaging often involves illumination and detection of a large portion of the substrate (1 cm^2) simultaneously. The ability to capture a relatively large field has the advantage of obviating the requirement for movable stages and optics, which reduces cost and simplifies instrument design. Another key difference between confocal scanners and CCD-based detection systems is that the latter often use continuous wavelength light sources such as arc lamps thereby obviating the need for multiple lasers. Fastidious filtering of emission spectra in CCD-based systems minimizes optical cross-talk between different channels. Detailed descriptions of both confocal scanners and CCD imaging systems are provided in Chapter 2.

Once the fluorescent emission from the microarrays is converted into a digital output by the detection system, the data files (usually 16-bit TIFF) are quantitated and interpreted. Quantitation is usually accomplished by superimposing a grid over the microarray image and computing an average intensity value for each microarray element with automated software. Intensity values can then be converted into biologically relevant outputs such as the number of mRNAs per cell, by comparing the experimental and controls elements present in a given microarray. Quantitative gene expression, genotyping, and other outputs are then correlated with the gene sequences represented in the microarray and higher order relationships such as co-regulation and gene regulatory networks can be identified. Quantitation and data mining software are described in detail in subsequent chapters (see Chapters 2–10).

4. Applications of microarrays

In a manner similar to the polymerase chain reaction (PCR), microarrays have a multitude of applications many of which will develop and evolve over time (21, 25, 29–31). Though the first application of biochips was in gene expression monitoring (9–17), the strategy of using an ordered array of biomolecules on a chip to examine a biochemical sample is generally applicable (*Figure 1*). In addition to gene expression analysis, hybridization-based assays have been used for mutation detection (28, 32–36), polymorphism analysis (2), mapping (37), evolutionary studies (40), and other applications (38, 39). Microarray assays could also be used to monitor the binding of proteins to nucleic acids, small molecules, and other proteins, but these applications have yet to be developed.

Hybridization analysis of genomic DNA can identify single base changes, deletions, and insertions in both coding and non-coding DNA. Hybridization analysis of DNA can also be used to measure the amount of a DNA sequence present, which is important in establishing gene copy number and chromosomal ploidy. In principle, *de novo* sequencing on chips is also feasible but has yet to be demonstrated.

Samples for DNA analysis can obtained either from total genomic DNA or from cloned fragments, by enzymatic incorporation of fluorescent nucleotides. Fluorescent DNA samples can also be obtained by PCR amplification with fluorescent primer pairs. RNA copies of DNA can also be used to examine cloned DNA fragments. RNA probes are usually prepared from cloned DNA by the incorporation of fluorescent nucleotides with RNA polymerase.

Hybridization analysis of RNA can provide information about which genes are expressed in a given sample and at what level. In gene expression applications, fluorescent probes are usually prepared from RNA by enzymatic incorporation of fluorescent nucleotides into complementary DNA (cDNA) by the use of reverse transcriptase. RNA probes for expression monitoring can also be made by linear amplification of cloned cDNA with RNA polymerase (see Chapter 7). In experiments with cDNA microarrays where the hybridization temperatures are sufficient to remove secondary structure in the DNA, a mixture of intact single-stranded molecules (300–3000 nt) provide robust hybridization signals. For assays involving microarrays of oligonucleotides where hybridization temperatures are generally lower, intense hybridization typically requires reducing the size of the molecules in the probe mixture into smaller (50–100 nt) fragments. Nucleic acid size reduction can be accomplished by both chemical (11, 16, 28, 40) and enzymatic means (2).

Unlike DNA and RNA analysis, the use of biochips to explore parallel protein function has proven much more difficult to implement. One shortcoming derives from the fact that many protein–protein interactions, unlike hybridization reactions which involve the interactions of linear sequences, occur with polypeptide surfaces that result from folded, three-dimensional amino acid sequences. The requirement for folded proteins in microarray assays is problematic for several reasons. First, microarray fabrication would have to be implemented in such a way as to maintain the delicate, folded properties of the proteins. The use of harsh chemicals, heat, drying, and the like in protein chip fabrication would compromise the quality of the microarray. Secondly, interactions between folded proteins display a much greater sequence-dependency than hybridization reactions. Sequence-dependency of the interactions inherently complicate reaction kinetics and assay quantitation. Thirdly, the preparation of high quality, fluorescent protein samples remains to be achieved. These and other problems have slowed the implementation of protein microarray technology.

5. Chips and pharmacogenomics

One exciting application of microarray technology is in the area of pharmacogenomics, a new field in biomedicine focused at the interface between pharmacology and genomics (*Table 4*). Pharmacology is the branch of science that endeavours to understand the preparation, use, and effects of drugs. Genomics endeavours to provide the complete sequence of genomes, and a complete knowledge of genes and gene functions. The two disciplines are complementary and synergistic in several respects (*Table 4*).

The complete sequence of all of the genes in a genome provides, by definition, a sequence of all of the gene products encoded by the genome. Because most drugs act at the protein level to disrupt or alter protein function, a complete genomic sequence provides all of the potential drug targets for a given

Table 4. Microarrays in pharmacogenomics

Application	Gene expression	Sequence analysis
Mechanism of drug action	Altered expression patterns provide clues to drug function	Re-sequencing can map site of protein–drug interaction
Lead compound identification	Can superimpose altered expression pattern in disease state with effect of small molecule	Can use genotyping data to guide lead compound identification
Lead compound optimization	Can screen for lead with largest effect on expression	Can correlate genotype data with lead compound activity
Toxicity	Secondary changes in expression can inform mechanism of toxicity	Can correlate toxicity with genotype to identify genes
Turnover	Expression changes can inform pharmacodynamics	Can correlate turnover with genotype
Efficacy	Expression differences among individuals can determine efficacy	Polymorphic differences among individuals can determine efficacy

organism. Pharmacogenomics thus derives tremendous benefit from having a complete list of all possible drug targets in advance of initiating the drug discovery process.

The central role of microarray technology in functional genomics (25, 30, 31) suggests an important role of chips in pharmacogenomics. Microarrays allow rapid gene expression monitoring and sequence analysis at the genomic level. This information will have an impact on many aspects of the drug discovery process (*Table 4*). Many drugs probably exert specific effects on gene expression that correlate with the mode of action of a given drug. Microarray-based analysis of gene expression at the genomic level should therefore prove useful in understanding the mechanistic basis of action of many drugs.

A growing body of evidence suggests that changes in gene expression may correlate with the onset of a given human disease (8–12). Chip-based analysis of disease tissues should allow the identification of genes whose expression is altered in a given illness. Many small molecules may also alter gene expression at a global level. It might therefore be possible to superimpose altered expression in a disease state, and with the changes that result from treatment with a small molecule to gain valuable information about classes of molecules that may be effective in combating a given disease (*Table 4*). The expected interplay of the genome and drug development suggests a role for microarrays in many additional aspects of pharmacogenomics including lead compound screening and optimization, toxicity, pharmacodynamics, and drug efficacy (*Table 4*). Microarray data, coupled with clinical information, promise to accelerate and reduce the cost of drug development.

14

6. Summary

Genomic information determines the form and function of an organism. Genes, the fundamental functional units of the genome, encode proteins which execute the genomic instructions. Biological differences among individuals in a population are due to both genetic and environmental factors. These influences can be understood by studying variability in genomic sequence (mutations and polymorphisms) and in how much of each gene product is made in a given cell or tissue (gene expression). By providing massive, parallel platforms for data gathering, microarray assays represent a fundamental technical advance in biomedical research. Biochips enable the use of advanced fabrication, detection, and data mining technologies which allow data gathering at an unprecedented rate. One of the many exciting applications of microarrays is in pharmacogenomics, the fusion of genome research and drug discovery.

References

1. Marmur, J. and Lane, D. (1960). *Proc. Natl. Acad. Sci. USA*, **46**, 453.
2. Wang, D. G., Fan, J. B., Siao, C. J., Berno, A., Young, P., Sapolsky, R., *et al.* (1998). *Science*, **280**, 1077.
3. Fleischmann, R. D., Adams, M. D., White, O., Clayton, R. A., Kirkness, E. F., Kerlavage, A. R., *et al.* (1995). *Science*, **269**, 496.
4. Fields, C., Adams, M. D., White, O., and Venter, J. C. (1994). *Nature Genet.*, **7**, 345.
5. Johnston, M., Hillier, L., Riles, L., Albermann, K., Andrè, B., Ansorge, W., *et al.* (1997). *Nature*, **387**, 87.
6. Schena, M. and Davis, R. W. (1998). In *PCR methods manual* (ed. M. Innis, D. Gelfand, and J. Sninsky), pp. 445–55. Academic Press, San Diego.
7. Yamamoto, K. R. (1985). *Annu. Rev. Genet.*, **19**, 209.
8. Schena, M. (1996). *Bioessays*, **18**, 427.
9. Schena, M., Shalon, D., Davis, R. W., and Brown, P. O. (1995). *Science*, **270**, 467.
10. Schena, M., Shalon, D., Heller, R., Chai, A., Brown, P. O., and Davis, R. W. (1996). *Proc. Natl. Acad. Sci. USA*, **93**, 10614.
11. Lockhart, D. J., Dong, H., Byrne, M. C., Follettie, M. T., Gallo, M. V., Chee, M. S., *et al.* (1996). *Nature Biotechnol.*, **14**, 1675.
12. DeRisi, J., Penland, L., Brown, P. O., Bittner, M. L., Meltzer, P. S., Ray, M., *et al.* (1996). *Nature Genet.*, **14**, 457.
13. Heller, R. A., Schena, M., Chai, A., Shalon, D., Bedilion, T., Gilmore, J., *et al.* (1997). *Proc. Natl. Acad. Sci. USA*, **94**, 2150.
14. DeRisi, J. L., Iyer, V. R., and Brown, P. O. (1997). *Science*, **278**, 680.
15. Lashkari, D. A., DeRisi, J. L., McCusker, J. H., Namath, A. F., Gentile, C., Hwang, S. Y., *et al.* (1997). *Proc. Natl. Acad. Sci. USA*, **94**, 13057.
16. Wodicka, L., Dong, H., Mittmann, M., Ho, M.-H., and Lockhart, D. J. (1997). *Nature Biotechnol.*, **15**, 1359.
17. de Saizieu, A., Certa, U., Warrington, J., Gray, C., Keck, W., and Mous, J. (1998). *Nature Biotechnol.*, **16**, 45.

18. Grunstein, M. and Hogness, D. S. (1975). *Proc. Natl. Acad. Sci. USA*, **72**, 3961.
19. Benton, W. D. and Davis, R. W. (1977). *Science*, **196**, 180.
20. Shalon, D., Smith, S. J., and Brown, P. O. (1996). *Genome Res.*, **6**, 639.
21. Lemieux, B., Aharoni, A., and Schena, M. (1998). *Mol. Breeding*, **4**, 277.
22. Fodor, S. P. A., Read, J. L., Pirrung, M. C., Stryer, L., Tsai Lu, A., and Solas, D. (1991). *Science*, **251**, 767.
23. Blachard, A. (1998). In *Genetic engineering, principles and methods* (ed. J. Setlow), Vol. 20. Plenum Press.
24. Khrapko, K. R., Khorlin, A. A., Ivanov, I. B., Chernov, B. K., Lysov, Yu. P., Vasilenko, S. K., *et al.* (1991). *Mol. Biol.*, **25**, 581.
25. Schena, M., Heller, R. A., Theriault, T. P., Konrad, K., Lachenmeier, E., and Davis, R. W. (1998). *Trends Biotechnol.*, **16**, 301.
26. Sosnowski, R. G., Tu, E., Butler, W. F., OíConnell, J. P., and Heller, M. J. (1997). *Proc. Natl. Acad. Sci. USA*, **94**, 1119.
27. Kallioniemi, A., Kallioniemi, O. P., Sudar, D., Rutovitz, D., Gray, J. W., Waldman, F., *et al.* (1992). *Science*, **258**, 818.
28. Chee, M., Yang, R., Hubbell, E., Berno, A., Huang, X. C., Stern, D., *et al.* (1996). *Science*, **274**, 610.
29. Southern, E. M. (1996). *Trends Genet.*, **12**, 110.
30. Hoheisel, J. D. (1997). *Trends Biotechnol.*, **15**, 465.
31. Fodor, S. P. A. (1997). *Science*, **277**, 393.
32. Cronin, M. T., Fucini, R. V., Kim, S. M., Masino, R. S., Wespi, R. M., and Miyada, C. G. (1996). *Hum. Mutat.*, **7**, 244.
33. Hacia, J. G., Brody, L. C., Chee, M. S., Fodor, S. P. A., and Collins, F. S. (1996). *Nature Genet.*, **14**, 441.
34. Kozal, M. J., Shah, N., Shen, N., Yang, R., Fucini, R., Merigan, T. C., *et al.* (1996). *Nature Med.*, **2**, 793.
35. Drmanac, S., Kita, D., Labat, I., Hauser, B., Schmidt, C., Burczak, J. D., *et al.* (1998). *Nature Biotechnol.*, **16**, 54.
36. Hacia, J. G., Makalowski, W., Edgemon, K., Erdos, M. R., Robbins, C. M., Fodor, S. P., *et al.* (1998). *Nature Genet.*, **18**, 155.
37. Sapolsky, R. J. and Lipshutz, R. J. (1996). *Genomics*, **33**, 445.
38. Shoemaker, D. D., Lashkari, D. A., Morris, D., Mittmann, M., and Davis, R. W. (1996). *Nature Genet.*, **14**, 450.
39. Cheung, V. G., Gregg, J. P., Gogolin-Ewens, K. J., Bandong, J., Stanley, C. A., Baker, L., *et al.* (1998). *Nature Genet.*, **18**, 225.
40. Hacia, J. G., Makalowski, W., Edgemon, K., Erdos, M. R., Robbins, C. M., Fodor, S. P., *et al.* (1998). *Nature Genet.*, **18**, 155.

2

Confocal scanning microscopy in microarray detection

MACK J. SCHERMER

1. Introduction: microarrays, fluorescence, and detection

All microarrays require fluorescence scanning to extract their experimental results. The confocal laser scanner delivers the highest image and data quality, a significant performance advantage. This chapter will describe the scanning process from an instrument point of view. It is divided into three parts. Sections 1 and 2 will describe the relevant characteristics of microarrays and all types of microarray scanners. Sections 3–7 will describe the design options and critical characteristics of confocal scanners. Finally, Section 8 will describe one commercial confocal implementation, the ScanArray®.

1.1 Detection characteristics of microarrays

This section will describe the aspects of microarrays that are most relevant from the point of view of a scanning instrument. Microarrays consist of small samples of DNA or other biological matter arranged on a flat surface. The DNA or other material is tagged with a fluorescent probe so that a fluorescence measurement will reveal the concentration of the sample, with a typical fluorescence dynamic range of between about 400:1 and 4000:1 limited by background fluorescence. The flat substrate is generally made of chemically treated glass, and is often in the form of a 25 mm × 75 mm microscope slide. Microarrays are described at length in several other chapters; this chapter will confine itself to the aspects of microarrays related to fluorescence detection.

Many DNA arrays incorporate samples tagged with multiple fluorescent probes, most often two. In the example of differential gene expression testing one probe is the control (normal tissue, for example) and the other probe represents the test (diseased tissue). The sample is scanned at two wavelengths, and the ratio of the fluorescence emissions of the two wavelengths represents the differential gene expression. This ratiometric approach reduces the need for absolute calibration of the sample preparation process. Array scanners generally require at least two different 'channels', or detection wavelengths.

A microarray consists of 'dots' and 'background', where the dots are the samples and the background is all of the area between the dots. While the substrate of the array is glass, the dots actually bind to chemical surface treatment on the surface of the glass. Surface treatments are used here to provide chemical binding affinity to the DNA samples and to produce very high surface tension. High surface tension prevents the liquid droplet of sample from spreading out when the array is made, helping to keep the dot size small and uniform, allowing increased density of the dots.

Microarray fluorescence data analysis almost always compares the fluorescent intensity of each dot to the local background around the dot. The substrate's surface treatment can degrade the scanning results if it fluoresces measurably in the wavelength ranges of interest and increases the fluorescence background level.

Dots may be anywhere from 25–500 μm in diameter. As of this writing, most DNA microarray dots are 100 μm $\pm$ 50 μm diameter, with the trend toward the smaller sizes. The dots are formed by small droplets of liquid drying in place on the substrate. Dot diameter variation affects scanning results. Scanners detect the area concentration of fluorescent dye; a droplet that spreads more than its otherwise identical neighbour will have a lower area concentration of dye, and will produce a scan signal that is inversely proportional to the dot area.

Contamination of the array by dust or almost any material can also affect scanning results adversely. All organic materials fluoresce. Microarray scanners that are sufficiently sensitive for the application will also clearly detect common airborne dust particles (e.g. clothing fibres, skin, finger oil).

Dry spotted microarray dots are quite thin, usually less than 10 μm. This thinness allows the use of the confocal scanning approach. Confocal scanning (described in Section 3) deliberately limits the depth of focus of the scanner, which prevents the imaging of many undesired background artefacts. Fluorescent dust, contamination on the back surface of the sample, fluorescence of the glass substrate itself, and fluorescence contamination from any of the scanner's internal optical components which may be 'glowing' in the field of view are all strongly attenuated by the confocal approach.

There may be significant variations in the fluorescence signal intensities between arrays, often due to minor differences in dye incorporation during reverse transcription and subsequent hybridization yields during microarray sample preparation. Microarray scanners need to have a sensitivity adjustment range that probably far exceeds the dynamic range of measurement of any one sample. A sensitivity adjustment range of at least 10000:1 is required for a general purpose instrument.

1.2 A brief description of fluorescence

Fluorescence in biological detection is a broad topic that has been described more comprehensively elsewhere (1). A brief description highlighting the aspects most relevant to microarray scanning is offered here.

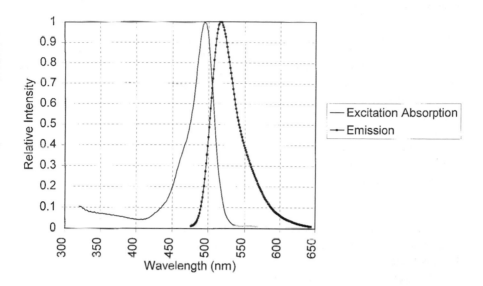

Figure 1. The relative excitation efficiency versus wavelength, or excitation absorption, for FITC (left-hand curve). The emission wavelength spectrum is also shown (right-hand curve) when the dye is excited at 400 nm.

Fluorescence light is emitted from a dye or fluorophore which is illuminated by excitation light. The fluorescence emission wavelength for the conventional fluorescence used in microarrays is always longer than the wavelength of the excitation light. Each dye has a curve describing the efficiency of excitation versus wavelength; an example curve for FITC (fluorescein isothiocyanate, a common dye used in microarrays) is shown in *Figure 1*.

This graph shows an excitation curve with a peak at 494 nm and fairly steep slopes away from both sides of the peak. The emission curve peaks at 518 nm. The wavelength difference between the emission and excitation peaks is 24 nm, which is typical for most dyes used in microarrays. This wavelength difference between the two peaks is called the Stokes shift.

Graphs such as these can be misleading at first look. This one suggests that, for example, that FITC can be excited at 510 nm, and produce some fraction of the fluorescence emission in the 475–510 nm range. That is not so; the emission is always at a longer wavelength than the excitation. The excitation curve and emission curves on this graph were not produced simultaneously. They are in fact very different sets of data placed on the same numerical grid for convenience of display.

The excitation curve is generated by measuring fluorescence emission at a single, long wavelength while the excitation wavelength is varied. The emission is measured at a wavelength longer than the longest excitation wavelength intended to be characterized. In *Figure 1*, the fluorescence was measured at 600 nm while the excitation was varied to generate the excitation curve

The emission curve is generated by measuring the intensities of narrow bands of fluorescence at many different wavelengths while keeping the excitation wavelength constant. The excitation wavelength used is shorter than the shortest emission wavelength intended to be measured; it was about 350 nm in the case illustrated in *Figure 1*. The emission curve is a true spectrum. The emitted light is not all at one wavelength but is distributed about a peak.

Reading such a graph allows the microarray scanner designer to specify wavelength selection components appropriate for the given dye. Excitation light should be provided at a wavelength that provides reasonably efficient excitation, at least at the 50–70% level. The excitation wavelength cannot be too close to the emission peak or it will pollute the fluorescence signal, so it needs to be on the left side of the excitation peak. For FITC, that suggests excitation wavelengths between about 470–495 nm.

Fluorescence is generally linear, such that the power of the emission light is directly proportional to the power of the excitation light. This process breaks down at high levels of excitation where the fluorescence output saturates or the dye is damaged by the incoming photons. Also, the fluorescence emission is typically orders of magnitude weaker than the excitation light in microarray applications.

The final aspect of fluorescence emission that is relevant to microarray scanners is that the emission from a dye molecule is spherical. Each dye molecule absorbs excitation photons and emits fluorescence photons. The emitted photon can go in any direction, with no directional preference relative to the incoming light. A fluorescence detecting instrument must therefore gather in the emission light from some fraction of this sphere. As microarray scanning utilizes very low levels of emission, this geometric fact is a major driver of the instrument design.

1.3 Optical requirements of a detection instrument

Microarray scanners can take many forms, whether confocal or not, but any of these instruments must provide the following functions:

- excitation
- emission light collection
- spatial addressing
- excitation/emission discrimination
- detection

1.3.1 Excitation

Excitation light can be generated by a variety of sources, such as lasers, arc or filament lamps, or LEDs. Excitation must be limited in its wavelength so that it does not overlap the emission, so broadband emitters such as lamps and LEDs require filters to select the excitation spectral band. Lasers generally produce light at a single, well-known wavelength (with some complications in diode lasers) and may not require excitation filtering. Lamp sources can be used to provide multiple excitation wavelengths with the simple addition of an excitation filter changer or other wavelength tuner. Multiple lasers are required in instruments delivering multiple laser excitation wavelengths. The function is sometimes provided by a multi-wavelength laser (also called multi-line; laser wavelengths are referred to as laser lines), but these tend to be more awkward and expensive than multiple lasers.

The excitation light must be directed onto the microarray sample. This can be done in a flood illumination manner, where a large area of the sample is excited at one time. Flood illumination is most often used with CCD camera type instruments and is infrequently used with confocal scanners. Non-uniformity of flood illumination across the excitation area on the sample is a concern that the instrument designer must address when using this method.

Alternatively, the excitation light may be focused to a small spot to illuminate a very small portion of the sample. This choice is tied in with light gathering and spatial addressing, described below. Focused spot illumination provides very intense excitation (up to $10\,000$ watt/cm^2 or more in microarray scanners) for a very short time on a given area as the spot scans across the sample.

Excitation wavelengths are chosen based on the intended dyes, as described in Section 1.2. The wavelength should be on the left side of the dye's excitation peak, but still in the range where the excitation efficiency is good. The lower the excitation efficiency, the more excitation light must be delivered to the sample to provide a given level of fluorescence. Excessive excitation light is not desirable; it can either damage the sample through photobleaching or pollute the fluorescence emission signal, which is much lower in intensity.

1.3.2 Light collection

The fluorescence light is most often gathered or collected with an objective lens. This is a lens that focuses on the sample and directs all emitted light within some angular range or cone into a detection path. The size of the solid angle of collection is critical. As the fluorescence emission is spherical, the fraction of the sphere that is intercepted by the objective lens is the first determinant of the light gathering efficiency of the instrument. The light collection angle of a lens is most often characterized by the numerical aperture (or NA). *Figure 2* is a plot of numerical aperture versus light collection efficiency for a point source spherical emitter.

An NA of 1.0 describes a lens that collects light over an entire hemisphere; this corresponds to a collection efficiency of 50%. Most confocal laser microarray scanners have NAs between 0.5–0.9, while most CCD-based array scanners have NAs between 0.2–0.5.

Still other array scanners do not use objective lenses. An integrating sphere

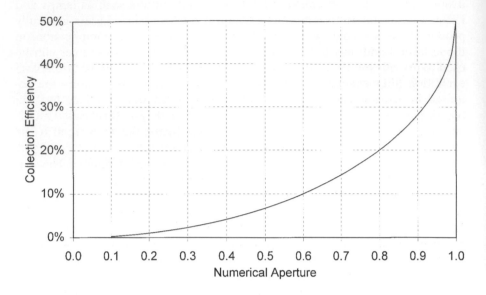

Figure 2. Collection efficiency of an objective lens at various NAs.

may be used to gather some fraction of the emission light, although with efficiency diminished from multiple reflections in the sphere (2). Yet another approach is to use no explicit light gathering element at all, and simply placing a detector with some area in a staring position over the sample. This arrangement's light collection efficiency is determined by the solid angle subtended by the detector compared to the sphere defined by the illuminated point on the sample. For example, some breadboard scanners utilize a bare 25 mm diameter detector about 100 mm from the excitation point, yielding an effective numerical aperture of 0.12.

1.3.3 Spatial addressing

Spatial addressing refers to measuring the fluorescence from small, specific areas on the sample. The sample is divided up into pixels, where each pixel is significantly smaller than a microarray dot. The spatial resolution must be finer than the dot size so that dot-edge artefacts and other non-uniformities can be accounted for in the quantification of the fluorescence signal. Scanners for 100 μm diameter microarray dots commonly use pixel sizes between 5–20 μm.

Spatial addressing is done either by using a multi-element detector array, such as a CCD, or by mechanical scanning. Most CCD cameras are configured to stare at an area that has been flood illuminated, and provide an image divided into pixels directly by the CCD detector. The limitations to this approach are the generally smaller NA lenses accommodated by CCD detectors and the cost of the back-illuminated, actively cooled CCD elements, and cross-talk between pixels due to optical scatter.

Mechanical scanning involves focusing the excitation beam to a point about the size of a pixel, and collecting emissions from just that small area with a single element detector. To cover the area of the sample, motion or scanning is required. This can be done by scanning the beams with mirrors (3), moving the sample, or a combination of both. Scanning adds considerable mechanical complexity to the system compared to a CCD camera system, but allows the use of higher NA light collection optics, higher spatial selectivity, and less expensive detectors. In low light applications, the higher optical collection efficiency is paramount.

1.3.4 Excitation/emission discrimination

Microarray fluorescence emission power is typically several orders of magnitude less intense than the excitation power. In order to detect the small fluorescence signal without a large contribution from the excitation light, some optical means must be incorporated into a microarray scanner to separate the two types of light. Since the beams are at different wavelengths, wavelength separation is the primary means, although specific geometric arrangements contribute as well.

Most objective lens-based microarray scanners use epi-illumination, where the excitation and emission beams follow the same path through the objective lens to and from the sample, but in opposite directions. This arrangement allows reflections and scatter from the sample to mix with the fluorescence beam. A beamsplitter element is used as the first separator of these beams.

One type of beamsplitter is a colour separating dichroic or multichroic interference filter, which reflects the excitation beam and transmits the emission beam at a slightly longer wavelength. These are commonly available, and can work well with one, two, or three different excitation/emission wavelength pairs. With four or more wavelengths, it is difficult to design and make a single multichroic beamsplitter with good performance at each colour.

A different type of beamsplitter is a geometric beamsplitter, shown in *Figure 3*. In scanning systems with an objective lens NA above about 0.6 and approximately 10 μm pixel size, the excitation beam is much smaller in diameter than the emission beam upstream of the objective lens. A small mirror, which reflects the laser beam but passes the bulk of the emission beam in an annular section works well as a wavelength-independent beamsplitter.

A beamsplitter that worked perfectly would complete the excitation/emission separation task, but no beamsplitter works perfectly. Emission filters are typically placed in the emission beam before the detector. These are interference filters that pass a narrow band of wavelengths near the dye's emission peak, and block all other light including the excitation light. This second layer of discrimination is required in the microarray application.

Scanners are built without beamsplitters by placing the excitation and

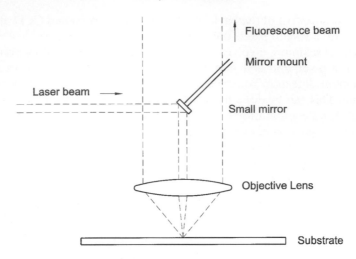

Figure 3. A geometric beamsplitter in an epi-illuminated scanner.

emission beam paths on different axes. This approach can work well for rejecting excitation light from the emission path, but it is difficult to implement with a high NA objective lens. Such lenses need to be placed very close to the sample, often less than 1 mm away, leaving little room for an excitation beam to enter from an angle.

Other types of components can be used for wavelength discrimination, such as prisms and gratings. These can offer some interesting features, such as continuous wavelength tunability. However, properly specified emission filters generally perform the best and most cost-effectively in microarray scanning due to the high excitation light rejection required.

1.3.5 Detection

The detector in a fluorescence scanner converts the low levels of light to an electrical signal. Detectors found in array scanners include photomultiplier tubes (PMTs), CCD arrays, and avalanche photodiodes (APDs). Each has advantages and disadvantages, and must be selected as part of the overall architecture of an instrument for a particular range of applications.

PMTs are the most sensitive detectors in the visible wavelength range. They are single point detectors and require a scanning system to provide spatial addressing of a microarray sample. It is convenient to change the PMT sensitivity by varying a control voltage, which provides at least part of the sensitivity adjustment range required in an array scanner. PMT sensitivity falls off rapidly between the red and near-IR, so their usefulness is generally limited to the visible range.

A CCD doesn't have the inherent low noise amplification of a PMT, and therefore usually needs more external amplification to reach the maximum sensitivity of a PMT. One major disadvantage is the difficulty in using a CCD detector with a high NA (0.6–0.9) collection system, limiting the optical signal available for detection. This is very important in dim light situations, as the statistics of the photon stream will ultimately determine the detection floor of the instrument. The other disadvantage is the impracticality of incorporating a CCD in a confocal system, the advantages of which are detailed in Section 3. In higher light applications, these disadvantages may be outweighed by the CCD detector array's built-in scanning mechanism.

2. Sample handling

Since all microarray scanners need to hold and locate the array substrate so that it is positioned properly with respect to the optics, this topic applies to all types of array scanners. This aspect of an instrument often requires precision positioning to maintain constant focus and image geometry from sample-to-sample. This section will mostly refer to microarray substrates that are glass microscope slides, which constitute the vast majority of spotted microarray substrates used today. Most of the considerations discussed apply equally to non-standard proprietary substrates as well.

2.1 'Standard' microscope slides

Microscope slides have become the *de facto* standard substrate for micro-arrays and dominate the market, but there is no single standard describing microscope slides. They are widely available in a variety of sizes, thicknesses, edge and corner configurations, and end treatment. *Table 1* summarizes the selection available from just one large American laboratory supplier, with some dimensions and tolerances. A general purpose scanning instrument needs to be able to accommodate the full range of slide types.

Table 1. Some characteristics of 'standard' microscopic slides

Slide type	'Inch': 1" × 3"	'Metric': 25 mm × 75 mm
X-Y dimensions, inches (mm)	1.0" × 3.0", ± 0.02" (25.4 mm × 76.2 mm, ± 0.5 mm)	0.98" × 2.95", ± 0.02" (25 mm × 76 mm, ± 0.5 mm)
Thickness dimensions	'Standard': 0.04" ± 0.002" (1.02 mm ± 0.05 mm) 'Thick': 0.047" ± 0.004" (1.2 mm ± 0.1 mm)	0.04" ± 0.002" (1.02 mm ± 0.05 mm)
Corners	Sharp, bevelled	Sharp, rounded
Edges	Sharp, bevelled	Sharp
Surface treatments on ends	Plain, sandblasted, painted; one or both sides	Plain, sandblasted, painted; one or both sides

---

Locating the sample by its top surface simplifies the accommodation of large thickness variations. The sample holder should allow easy loading and unloading of a sample, and may need to accommodate an autoloading accessory for high volume scanning. The materials used in the sample holder must withstand the abrasion of thousands of insertions and removals.

2.2 Other formats

Other sample formats in development and limited use as microarray substrates include plastic slides, proprietary glass substrates of various shapes and sizes, and enclosed liquid-filled cells. Each requires specific sample holding solutions; for example, plastic is much less stiff than glass and more challenging to keep flat and in-focus in a confocal scanner. Liquid-filled cells require imaging through the glass to the second surface which typically requires a specific objective lens design as well as a custom sample holder.

2.3 Sample environment

Most microarrays are scanned at room temperature in the dry state, with the dots dried on the surface of the substrate. Some popular dyes, FITC for example, emit stronger fluorescence in a wet state. This condition is produced in a scanner by wetting the array with the proper buffer solution and covering it with a thin cover glass. The sample holder must accommodate the full range of coverslip sizes to be useful in these applications. The scanner then scans through the cover glass.

Some researchers are investigating the scanning of arrays while controlling and varying the temperature while scanning to reveal additional information about the sample. At this writing, this capability is not available in any commercial scanning instrument.

3. Confocal scanning of microarrays

The above sections were a preamble to the main topic, which is the 'how' and 'why' of confocal scanning. This section will describe the confocal scanner optical arrangement, showing how the confocal arrangement blocks out many unwanted image artefacts, and discuss its advantages and disadvantages.

3.1 The confocal arrangement

With the above background in place, this section will illustrate the confocal scanning architecture and discuss its tradeoffs. As the name implies, confocal scanners have two focal points configured to limit the field of view in three dimensions. This limits light gathering from all locations outside of a small volume and rejects a variety of image artefacts. Confocal systems by definition image only a very small area (effectively one point; one pixel) and require scanning to acquire a multi-point image from a two-dimensional surface.

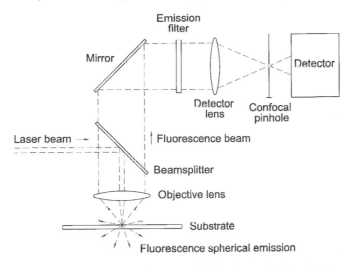

Figure 4. The confocal scanning arrangement in a microarray scanner.

The confocal optical arrangement shown in *Figure 4* operates as follows. The collimated (or parallel) laser beam is reflected from the beamsplitter into the objective lens. The laser beam fills only a fraction of the lens; how much depends on the particular choice of lens NA and the desired pixel size. The laser beam is focused on the sample, where it induces spherical fluorescence in all directions. The excitation beam also reflects back up toward the detector.

The objective lens collects a fraction of the spherical fluorescence emission and collimates it into a parallel beam. It also collects the reflected laser light, which is three to seven orders of magnitude more intense than the fluorescence. This return beam is again directed to the beamsplitter, which reflects most of the laser light back toward the laser source, and transmits most of the fluorescence beam up toward the detector. A mirror then folds the system without any optical functionality, followed by the emission filter which selects a narrow band of fluorescence emission and rejects all remaining laser excitation light.

The confocal nature of the system is embodied in the detector lens and the pin-hole. The detector lens focuses the collimated fluorescence beam to a small diameter, and a pin-hole is placed to allow passage of that focused beam and block all other light. This has the effect of restricting the depth of focus of the objective lens. A look at the path of an out-of-focus image through *Figure 5* reveals this.

A second point source of light below the focus on the sample, caused by a piece of dust for example, would emit light that also enters the objective lens. Since this second point is not at the objective lens' focus, however, the fluorescence beam travelling up toward the detector is not collimated (parallel), it

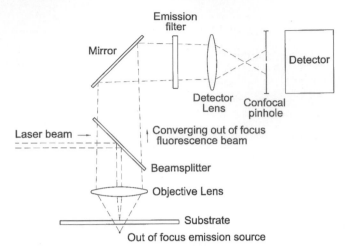

Figure 5. Emission light from an out-of-focus image point is blocked by the confocal pin-hole.

is converging. When this converging beam passes through the detector lens, it forms a focus in front of the pin-hole instead of at the pin-hole. The beam expands after the focus and has a large diameter where it strikes the pin-hole. This causes the pin-hole to reject most of the out-of-focus light. The same pin-hole rejection effect happens with light sources above the objective's focus. Only light from a narrow depth of focus at the sample can pass through the pin-hole efficiently.

3.2 Advantages and disadvantages of the confocal arrangement

In a microarray scanner, this restricted depth of focus strongly reduces the imaging of artefacts on the sample, such as dust and rear-surface reflections from the substrate. It also nearly eliminates the instrument's sensitivity to unintended fluorescence of components within the instrument, such as filters or the sample holder. In practice, it produces microarray images and data with dot-to-background (signal-to-noise) ratios far superior to non-confocal instruments.

The chief disadvantage of the confocal system is also the restricted depth of focus. It requires the scanning motion that generates the image to be performed with a deviation from flatness that is much less than the depth of focus, on the order of $\pm$ 10 μm. In systems where the beam is scanned, the field-flattening or F-theta scan lens must produce a very flat field. In all systems, scanning beam or moving substrate, the substrate must be kept flat and the substrate motion must also be kept flat. This complicates the mechanical and optical design but is the preferred path to maximum image quality.

3.3 Confocal implementations and tradeoffs

The confocal arrangement as shown in *Figure 4* is appropriate for a moving-substrate scanner. The arrangement can be implemented in a moving-beam scanner by inserting a scanning mirror between the beamsplitter and the objective lens (as in ref. 3), and making the objective lens a flat-field scan lens. A scan lens accepts a beam scanning through various angles and focuses it along a flat, straight line. Such lenses that can scan the width of a microscope slide are quite complicated and are generally limited to a NA of about 0.3 or less.

Simple objective lenses and much higher light collection efficiencies can be obtained with moving-lens or moving-substrate systems. A moving-substrate instrument moves the substrate in a raster fashion under the stationary optical system. A moving-lens system moves an entire optical head over a stationary substrate. The tradeoff is that these systems with larger moving masses typically have lower maximum scanning speeds than moving-beam systems. However, the high scanning speeds of a moving-beam system may not be usable in dim light situations where the statistics of photon detection determine the detection floor, so the gaining of potential scanning speed with the reduction of light collection efficiency can be self-defeating. Kain *et al.* (4) describe a moving-lens system, and Section 8 describes a moving-substrate system which takes advantage of the simple lens with high NA.

4. Wavelength discrimination: minimizing the background image

This section will describe in greater detail the instrument design criteria and tradeoffs involved in wavelength discrimination, or separating the desired fluorescence light from all of the other light before detection and quantification. The usefulness of the instrument to a bioresearcher hinges on this capability to a large extent. While the principles outlined here apply to all types of fluorescence scanners, the most desirable implementations for maximizing image quality can only be implemented in the laser confocal type.

Useful microarray scanners must detect very low levels of fluorescence light, in the picowatt range. At this low level, almost all materials fluoresce: the glass substrate, the chemicals comprising the substrate's surface coating, sample washing chemicals, lenses, filters, even DNA itself. The scanning instrument needs to maximize detection of the target dye's emission while minimizing detection of all of these other fluorescence sources. In addition, the reflected and scattered laser light, which is about one million times brighter than the dim fluorescence light from the microarray, must be rejected as well. Failure to separate the dye emission light properly from all of the competing sources results in a high background signal level. This background signal can define the dye concentration detection floor of the scanner and needs to be minimized.

4.1 Beamsplitter

All confocal scanners have some type of beamsplitter, as shown in *Figure 4*. This component must separate out the returning beam from the sample from the excitation beam. The glass sample substrate reflects about 4% of the laser light from the first surface. Some researchers are investigating the use of mirrored sample substrates to increase the fluorescence returned back up the optical path. A mirrored substrate reflects nearly all of the laser light.

The beamsplitter should reject most of the reflected laser light from the detection path while passing most of the fluorescence. A common component used for this is a dichroic or multichroic interference filter. These components commonly exhibit reflectance of over 90% for one, two, or three laser lines, and transmission in the 60–85% range for one, two, or three fluorescence bands. The 90% laser line reflection eliminates all but 10% of the laser reflection from the detector path. These components work adequately in many applications, but become increasingly difficult to implement with larger numbers of laser and fluorescence wavelengths in the instrument.

A geometric beamsplitter, such as the one illustrated in *Figure 3*, can show markedly improved performance over the dichroic type, with the added benefit of wavelength independence. Implementation of such a beamsplitter requires a number of instrument optical parameters to all be selected in concert. The primary assumption for the use of such a splitter is that the collimated excitation beam must be much smaller than the returning emission beam. This can only happen when the choice of focused excitation spot size and the focal length and NA of the objective lens allow it. In general, the technique works better with higher NAs. With an NA of 0.75, a focal length of 6.6 mm, and an input laser beam diameter of 0.75 mm, an objective lens aperture of 10 mm, and a focused excitation spot size of about 6 μm, the technique works quite well. The geometric splitter for this system can be constructed to transmit about 80% of the emission beam while rejecting almost all of the reflected laser light. This type of beamsplitter has been shown to increase the signal-to-background ratio on very dim samples by a factor of three over a dichroic splitter.

Other types of beamsplitters, such as polarizing beamsplitters and 50/50 broadband splitters, do not have sufficient excitation light rejection to be effective in microarray scanners.

4.2 Emission filters

The beamsplitter in a confocal microarray scanner is not adequate by itself for discriminating the fluorescent dye signal from the other light sources. As shown in *Figure 4*, an emission filter can be placed in the collimated emission beam prior to the confocal detector lens. An emission filter should transmit the desired wavelength band of the fluorescence signal and block all other light.

Examining, as an example, the fluorescence emission of FITC in *Figure 1*, the reader might conclude that the best emission filter would be one that includes most of the emission curve in its passband, say from 510–600 nm. This would deliver the maximum fluorescence light to the detector. In practice, the light in the emission beam is a more complicated mix. In addition to the dye's emission curve, there are several other emission curves competing with it: fluorescence of the glass substrate, the surface preparation chemicals, the sample washing chemicals, etc. These other 'noise' fluorescence curves are in general not defined and are variable. With that, the emission filter needs to maximize the dye signal while minimizing the competing fluorescence.

The best way to do that is to use a narrow band emission filter with the passband centred on the dye emission peak, as shown in *Figure 6*. This figure shows a filter passband that is 10 nm wide at its half-intensity points (FWHM). Passing the dye emission at its maximum intensity in a narrow window while blocking all light outside of the passband maximizes the signal-to-noise. The penalty for this approach is low throughput of the signal. The 10 nm FWHM, six cavity interference filters which have been found to provide optimum signal-to-noise performance typically have about 60% transmission at the peak, and as *Figure 6* shows, only a fraction of the total dye emission spectrum

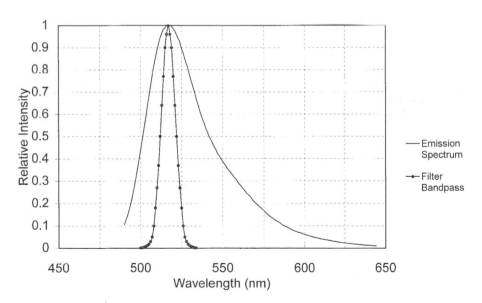

Figure 6. Pictorial superposition of a 10 nm FWHM bandpass emission filter on FITC emission.

overlaps the passband window. Such a filter will typically transmit 10–15% of the total dye emission.

The low optical throughput of a narrow band emission filter can only be tolerated in an instrument with high collection efficiency; e.g. a high NA objective lens. A microarray scanner with 10 nm FWHM emission filters centred on the dye peak works well with NAs above about 0.7. Filters with wider passbands increase background transmission more than signal transmission, and narrower filters simply bring signal and noise down together.

Emission filters also need to block the residual laser light not stopped by the beamsplitter. Conventional narrow band filters typically provide about 10^4 attenuation of the excitation wavelength 20–30 nm down from the dye's emission peak. Microarray detection performance is enhanced by greater attenuation at the specific laser wavelength. Either custom emission filters specified to block the laser line or separate laser blocker filters that increase laser attenuation to about 10^7 produce measurable performance gains.

5. Detectors

Confocal laser microarray scanners use PMTs as detectors almost universally. In spite of the apparent disadvantages of tubes (the need for high voltage, large unit-to-unit variation in sensitivity, larger size than photodiodes), the advantages dominate in most visible light microarray scanning applications.

A PMT can detect a single photon, or a beam of light that is so low in power that it is a series of photon events rather than a continuous power flux. The amplification built into the PMT amplifies the photon events into electron events with amplification factors of about one million, producing a low noise current which is straightforward to filter, integrate, and quantify using conventional instrumentation electronics. In addition, the PMT sensitivity or gain can be adjusted through a range of several hundred to one by varying the tube high voltage input. This built-in wide range of adjustment is ideal for microarray scanning where variations in the sample preparation process dictate that requirement in the instrument.

Conventional silicon detectors, such as PIN photodiodes, don't have the built-in low noise gain of a PMT, and also have significantly lower quantum efficiencies in the visible wavelength range. Thus, they require external amplification of several million to reach the equivalent light-to-signal sensitivity. This external amplification adds noise, resulting in a lower signal-to-noise ratio. Silicon detectors have a wavelength response that is peaked in the 800–900 nm range, which makes them more attractive in the near-IR range. PMTs typically show peak sensitivity in the 500 nm range and start falling off rapidly beyond 650 nm.

Avalanche photodiodes (APDs) do have built-in, low noise gain similar to the PMT. However, they still provide much lower quantum efficiency in the visible range and lack the PMTs convenient sensitivity adjustment mechanism.

Researchers have used cooled avalanche photodiodes successfully in array scanners utilizing near-IR dyes, but PMTs are superior for the more common visible dyes.

6. Signal processing and instrument control

The previous sections have focused on sample handling and particularly on optics and detection. While these disciplines reside at the core of any microarray scanner, the instrument is not complete or of use to a bioresearcher without signal processing and means for controlling the scanner. This section will illustrate the control and processing functions required in a complete instrument.

6.1 Sensitivity range requirements

The fluorescent yield of any microarray sample is largely unknown until it is scanned. Sample preparation steps that have high variability include dye incorporation during reverse transcription and hybridization. Different types and batches of gene expression arrays using the same dyes can exhibit brightness differences of 1000:1 from one to another. Well prepared samples can exhibit dynamic range of fluorescence of up to about 4000:1 within the microarray. Since the dynamic range of most scanners spans from about 4000–16000, there isn't enough dynamic headroom to accommodate the widely varying samples without changing the instrument sensitivity.

Two techniques are used to adjust sensitivity. First, the excitation power can be varied, typically by using a variable laser attenuator. Excitation power can usually be varied over a range of at least 100:1. Secondly, the PMT sensitivity can be changed, also over a range of at least 100:1, by varying the high voltage input. Both techniques superimpose, so an instrument adjustment range of more than 10000:1 can be obtained by incorporating both. This is adequate for a general purpose instrument.

Using as much excitation power as possible without damaging the sample by photobleaching is generally desirable. More excitation power generates more fluorescence photons, generating a cleaner and statistically more robust signal at the beginning of the imaging chain. If a sample is to be scanned many times, the laser power may need to be dropped to lessen accumulated photon damage to it.

Since these instruments have such a large adjustment range, it can be difficult to find the proper operating point without many trial scans. An automatic routine in the instrument that sets the sensitivity to make the brightest image feature just short of instrument saturation saves the user a lot of time.

6.2 Signal averaging and sampling

The optical signal generated by the excited fluorescent dyes is processed for conversion into a sequence of digital values. The signal consists of a stream of random photon emission events that, when properly averaged, correlate to the area density of dye molecules. However, the photons are emitted randomly over the space within a pixel and over the time of sampling. Therefore, the scanning instrument averages both spatially and temporally.

The scanned region is divided into equally sized pixels. Confocal and other spot-illuminated instruments independently excite each pixel and the resulting emitted fluorescence is collected for detection. The laser spot acts as a moving spatial averaging mechanism since the emission from the total spot area is summed during detection.

The shape and size of the laser spot determine its averaging characteristics. The spot typically has a Gaussian intensity profile that results in the dye molecules illuminated by the centre of the spot to be more excited and to emit more, and therefore to be more heavily weighted in the averaging processes. The FWHM spot size is typically chosen to be equal to that of the pixel. Larger spots would tend to average pixels together and smaller spots would not include the complete pixel in the spatial averaging.

After the optical signal is detected and converted to an electrical signal by the PMT, it requires further processing before being converted to digital data. The electrical signal still contains the randomness associated with individual photon emission events over time. The digitization process can be considered instantaneous relative to pixel dwell time. Electronic filtering is used to average the photon emission events into a signal that represents the information contained in each pixel.

Typically a time averaging, low pass filter is employed that uses an exponentially decreasing weight for signal values prior to the instant of digital conversion. These filters produce an exponentially decaying signature when filtering a step function. The time constant of the filter—the time required for the filter to decay to about one-third of its initial value after a step change—is the parameter set for proper data conversion. In practice, the time constant is set between one- and two-thirds of a pixel period. Longer time constants tend to average pixels together. Shorter time constants will tend to allow single photon events to distort the final data.

6.3 Dark signal

The detection components produce a non-zero signal even in the absence of light. This is called the dark signal, and its contributors include the PMT as well as its subsequent amplifiers and other circuitry. To the extent that this signal is constant over the time of an image scan, it can be subtracted out of the signal, and then will not affect the dynamic range of the instrument. Components of the dark signal that vary during scanning do limit it.

6.4 Image acquisition, display, and storage

A confocal microarray scanner is intended to perform an area scan of a sample and provide a digital map of the fluorescent intensities of each pixel.

The scanning system, whether it moves the beam, or the sample, or some combination, must produce a raster scan over an area. For a general purpose instrument the scan area should be selectable, so that the user need not wait for the instrument to cover the entire sample when the area of interest is smaller than that. In addition, a preview high speed, low resolution scanning mode is desirable, scanning only every five lines or so just to find a small array in a large field quickly.

Digitization of the pixels should be at 16-bit intensity resolution. 16-bit is a convenient format for downstream processing and manipulation. As an image is being scanned, it should be displayed on a monitor for preliminary inspection to make sure the sample is the right one, the settings are correct, etc. Image display is most often done with the fluorescent intensity mapped into false colours so that the human eye can distinguish more discrete levels on the screen.

After the image is scanned, it is saved or transferred to another computer application for quantification or other post-processing. The 16-bit TIFF (tagged image file format; .tif) format is the *de facto* standard for transferring microarray images, although some proprietary systems use proprietary formats.

6.5 Control interface and automation

All of the above optical and electronic functions have the most value in the laboratory when the user doesn't need to think about them. The instrument becomes useful when it has a simple, complete, and intuitive user interface to control it, and when commonly used sequences are automated. Microarray scanners are always controlled from a computer console. The successful commercial scanners available today, which have been refined with a great deal of user feedback, utilize graphical user interfaces that allow a new user to become productive very quickly with very little training or reading of manuals. They also allow experienced users to maintain a high level of productivity with minimum distraction from details.

Automation is particularly valuable in saving time for the user in the following areas:

(a) Setting, saving, and recalling sets of scanning parameters for particular users and types of samples.

(b) Automatic scanning of the sample at two or more wavelengths, with automatic saving of the resulting image files.

(c) Automatic sensitivity setting on one channel (auto-ranging) by scanning at low resolution and automatically adjusting excitation and detector settings to maximize dynamic range.

(d) Automatic sensitivity setting on multiple channels, commonly called 'balancing the channels'.

(e) Automatic internal calibration of excitation power settings and detector sensitivity settings.

The scanner or its host computer should also provide multi-gigabyte data storage, network connectivity, and support for large capacity removable storage media.

7. Instrument performance measures

Microarray scanners are complex instruments, embodying a large number of parameters and specifications. This section outlines the most important performance measures that most likely determine the suitability of a particular instrument for an application.

7.1 Number of lasers and fluorescence channels

The number of available scanning wavelengths (colours, channels) is fundamental to the instrument. A single excitation laser may excite several dyes and be used with several emission filters. However, there will be significant 'cross-talk' between these multiple dyes if they are used on a single sample. Independent channels, ones for multiple dyes that can be used on a single sample, almost always require separate laser sources of different wavelengths. One exception to this is scanning done with energy transfer dyes, which utilize the emission from a first dye to stimulate a second dye; but this is outside of the mainstream of microarray scanning. Two or four fluorescence channels with two lasers are common in first generation scanners, and three or four lasers with up to 10 selectable fluorescence bands are available in second generation instruments.

7.2 Detectivity

Detectivity is the minimum dot fluorescent brightness that can be distinguished from the background when the sensitivity is set so that the brightest element of the sample produces an intensity level at the full scale. From an instrument point of view, its unit of measure would be the number of dye molecules per unit area (fluors/μm^2). Bioresearchers generally don't know what the dye density is, due to the sample process uncertainties, and view this measure from an application point of view, such as a threshold gene expression level. Detectivity is often characterized with specially made microarrays that incorporate dilution series: sequential array dots with systematically decreasing dye concentrations. The detectivity for that array preparation process is then defined by the dimmest dot in the dilution series that can be detected.

Either the sample or the instrument can place the limit on detectivity. If the sample preparation results in relatively high background fluorescence between the dots, the sample will be the limit. If the instrument injects noise into the signal that can't be subtracted out, at a level that exceeds the sample background, the instrument will be the limit.

7.3 Sensitivity

Sensitivity is the instrument's conversion efficiency of light power to a digital value at a particular wavelength. It is a measure of the 'gain' of the instrument. Unlike detectivity, sensitivity is not dependent on the characteristics of a particular sample. Sensitivity can limit detectivity only if the scan data from a sample is too dim when the excitation and detector are both adjusted to maximum values. More often, the maximum settings for the instrument are not used, as those settings produce saturated data values.

7.4 Cross-talk

When scanning samples with multiple dyes, cross-talk can occur. Cross-talk is the excitation and detection of a dye with the 'wrong' or unintended excitation wavelength and emission filter. In differential gene expression, cross-talk negatively distorts the expression ratio between the two channels. It is minimized by the use of narrow band emission filters centred on the dye peaks, with good attenuation of out of band wavelengths. It is most completely minimized by the selection of dyes and laser wavelengths which are sufficiently far apart (approximately 50 nm is a good rule of thumb) to allow proper filtering.

7.5 Resolution

The spatial resolution of a microarray scanner is usually expressed as a pixel size, with 5, 10, and 20 μm being common in commercial devices. It is important that each microarray dot be imaged into many pixels so that edge effects and other defects can be rejected at the quantification stage. As a rule of thumb, the pixel dimension should be no larger than 1/8 to 1/10 of the diameter of the smallest microarray dot to be imaged.

7.6 Field size

The field size, the area on the substrate that can be scanned, must match the array making process. The larger the scan area, the more dots that can be placed on each sample. Usually, a 1.0 to 1.5 mm border around the periphery of the slide is not used, as it may be chipped or not flat. Combined with the slide size tolerances outlined in *Table 1*, the maximum usable area is about 22 mm × 73 mm. Many commercial scanners only scan 60 mm in the long direction, assuming that the user will want a 15 mm 'handle' on the end of the slide for handling and labelling.

7.7 Uniformity

Uniformity is a measure of the consistency of fluorescence emission and detection across the field. Uniformity of light collection throughout the image field is of particular concern for confocal scanners. The confocal feature limits the depth of focus, often to just a few tens of microns. This means that deviations from flatness in the scanning motion or in the sample itself at this small level will result in non-uniformity of the image across the field. Increasing the depth of focus by enlarging the confocal pin-hole relaxes the sample flatness requirements, but at the expense of adding unwanted image artefacts. Confocal scanners, particularly the moving-sample type, do have an advantage over flood illumination scanners in the delivery of uniform excitation power throughout the field.

Most users seek a $\pm$ 10% scanner uniformity across the field. At this level, sample preparation effects dominate the overall uniformity result.

7.8 Image geometry

Requirements for the scanner's image geometry depend greatly upon the post-processing applied to the image data. Image size, X-Y orthogonality, and pixel placement linearity matter a great deal if the image quantification software applies a fixed grid to the scanned image and expects to find dots in the centre of each box. More sophisticated microarray image quantification software applies a dynamic grid, 'finding' each dot regardless of its placement. Obviously, great precision in scanning geometry is less valuable if the precision delivered by the instrument that places spots on the array is low.

Most users are satisfied with image size and linearity tolerances of $\pm$ 2%. Many second generation scanners far exceed that level of precision.

Random geometry errors can also be important. These are often called 'jitter', and are manifested as jagged vertical lines in the raster image. When the line-to-line non-repeatability of scanning exceeds a pixel, the dot image's edges become jagged. This can cause problems in quantification when there are only a few pixels per dot.

The registration of multiple images of the same sample scanned at different wavelengths is also worth noting. Post-processing software that 'finds' the dots and automatically constructs a grid on the image usually creates the grid on the image from one channel and then uses the same grid on the images from different channels. Most array scanners maintain registration between subsequent scans at one pixel or less, which is adequate.

7.9 Throughput

Once all of the above image measures are proven adequate, users often focus on how many samples can be scanned in a day. Throughput specifications are only meaningful when applied to a resolution, an image field size, and the number of channels to be scanned on each sample. Some CCD camera-based scanners exhibit very high throughput, but are several factors less effective in detectivity of dim samples than even first generation confocal scanners.

Throughput for multichannel scanning can be increased dramatically by incorporating colour separating beamsplitters in the emission path, multiple detectors, and multiple signal processing modules and scanning multiple colours simultaneously. However, this increases the scanner cost and complexity, especially for multiple wavelength instruments, and may increase optical cross-talk.

A typical specification for a first generation scanner scanning a single colour over a 20 mm × 60 mm field is 5–15 minutes at 10 μm resolution. Most second generation scanners are faster.

7.10 Superposition of signal sources

This is not a performance measure, but is an important concept that fits better at this point in the chapter than elsewhere.

The image viewed on the scanner's monitor or quantified by the post processing software is not a simple image of the dye fluorescence in the microarray's dots. It is the superposition of several images, only one of which is desired:

(a) The fluorescence of the target dye being scanned (which is desired).
(b) Photon statistical noise (really part of the image, but looks like noise).
(c) Fluorescence of the background, due to other chemicals and the glass (not desired).
(d) Laser light reflection (actually a reflection image of the sample, but not desired).
(e) Electronic noise (not desired).

One cannot determine the relative contributions of each by examining any one image or image data set by itself. The data set is just a collection of pixel brightnesses, and the A/D converter doesn't care what the source was. In evaluating a new instrument, a user needs to make sure that the instrument and the microarray preparation process work together to reveal results with the required accuracy.

8. ScanArray® confocal microarray scanners

GSI Lumonics has developed a product line of confocal microarray scanners called ScanArray®. As of this writing, hundreds of these instruments are in use in biotech and genomics laboratories around the world.

8.1 Importance of integration

The information provided in the above sections is sufficient to allow an experienced instrumentation engineer to build a breadboard microarray scanner. In fact, many laboratories have done just that, and many of those have published their instrument descriptions. However, a great deal of the value of a microarray scanner lies in its integration into a complete, compact, robust, reliable product. Most researchers don't want to build a complex instrument, they want to use it with confidence and not think about it. Commercial instruments, developed with the benefit of the user feedback that is required to develop image quality standards and software control features, best meet researchers' needs.

8.2 ScanArray® architecture

The ScanArray® is a bench-top, moving-substrate, stationary optics, multi-laser, confocal scanner. This architecture utilizes simple optics, has a large NA for high light collection efficiency, and is low in cost. The compact size conserves valuable laboratory space. To benefit from those features without sacrificing throughput, a great deal of development effort has resulted in a servo-controlled sample moving mechanism that can scan up to 20 lines/sec.

HeNe and argon lasers of various colours provide excitation. A geometric beamsplitter and specially designed emission filters minimize laser reflection. A single PMT detector allows scanning one colour at a time, but with minimum cross-talk.

User control is provided by a host PC, either dedicated to the instrument in the ScanArray® 3000 or via a network connection in the ScanArray® 5000. Running under Windows®-95, 98, or NT, the host software provides quick, intuitive operation with convenience and automation of many tasks. *Table 2*

Table 2. ScanArray® specifications

	ScanArray® 3000 series	ScanArray® 5000 series
Architecture	Moving substrate, epi-illuminated, stationary optics, multicolour, sequential scanning	Moving substrate, epi-illuminated, stationary optics, multicolour, sequential scanning
Numerical aperture (NA)	0.75	0.75
Substrate	All 'standard' 1" × 3" microscope slides	All 'standard' 1" × 3" microscope slides
Field size	22 mm × 60 mm max. or smaller	22 mm × 73 mm max. or smaller
Image uniformity	± 10% max. over full field	± 10% max. over full field
Scanning speed	6 lines/sec max. at full field	20 lines/sec. max at full field
Resolution settings	10 μm; 50 μm (preview scan)	5, 10, 20 μm; 30, 50 μm (preview scans)
Lasers	Two (543 and 633 nm)	Up to four (488, 514, 543, 594, 612, or 633 nm)
Emission channels	2	Up to 10
Host computer	Dedicated Pentium®/Windows® PC	Networked Pentium®/Windows® PC
Output data	16-bit TIFF (.tif), bitmap (.bmp)	16-bit TIFF (.tif), bitmap (.bmp)
Dimensions	25" long × 10.5" wide × 11.5" high	30" long × 15.5" wide × 13.5" high
Power input	95–250 VAC, 47–63 Hz	95–250 VAC, 47–63 Hz
Weight	35 lb	60–70 lb, depending on laser configuration

illustrates the most significant specifications. Detectivity and cross-talk are not specified here as they are functional specifications that depend upon the substrate being scanned, for which commercial standards don't exist as of this writing. Suitability for an application is best determined by a demonstration.

8.3 ScanArray® advantages

Compared to the other commercially available microarray scanners, the ScanArray® product exhibits several advantages. The high NA objective lens combined with application developed filtering provides detectivity that leads the industry. The simple optical architecture leads to a very compact

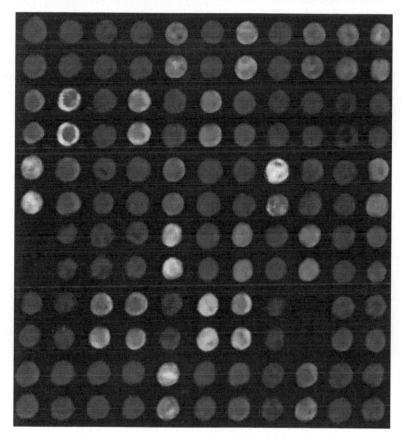

Figure 7. A small section of a fluorescence image from a gene expression array tagged with Cy3™. The dots are nominally 200 μm in diameter on 350 μm centre-to-centre spacing. This black and white representation does not reveal the range of fluorescent intensities to the eye as well as a false-colour image. Note the non-uniformity of intensities within some of the dots. Microarray quantification software will process this raw image data and produce a single value for each dot's intensity and local background value. This image was scanned by a ScanArray® 3000 instrument.

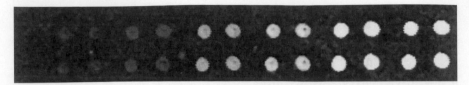

Figure 8. An example of a FITC dilution series used to test detectivity. Each group of four dots is a factor of four lower in concentration, moving right to left.

bench-top instrument with high reliability and low cost. Continuous collaboration with instrument users has resulted in a control interface that maximizes productivity with little training.

Microarray scanning instruments are complicated to compare. Many of the performance measures are interrelated and the selection criteria cannot be realistically narrowed down to a single specification; the entire instrument must be evaluated, often with a trial scan of the target samples. The specifications and features listed here were correct as of the time of writing. Features and upgrades are added periodically, so this description may not be current. *Figures 7* and *8* depict some greyscale microarray scanning results from ScanArray® instruments.

References

1. Ormerod, M. G. (ed.) (1994). In *Flow cytometry: a practical approach*, p. 29. IRL Press.
2. Tomei, L. D. (1988). US Patent 4 758 727.
3. Kain, R. C. (1998). US Patent 5 719 391.
4. Kain, R. C., Miller, M. F., and Majlof, L. (1996). US Patent 5 578 818.

3

Representational differences analysis and microarray hybridization for efficient cloning and screening of differentially expressed genes

STANLEY F. NELSON and CHRISTOPHER T. DENNY

1. Introduction

The determination of differential expression of genes between cell lines and tissues is a powerful tool in modern biological research. Several recent and rapid PCR-based methods including subtractive suppressive hybridization (SSH), representational difference analysis (RDA), and differential display (1–4), have been proposed for the cloning of genes which are differentially expressed between two tissues. These methods have been validated and successfully applied to specific problems (5–12). Recently, cDNA and oligonucleotide microarrays have been developed and used to quantitate differential gene expression by hybridizing a complex mRNA-derived probe onto an array of PCR products or oligonucleotides representing specific cDNAs (13–15). Microarrays allow thousands of genes to be monitored simultaneously for expression level and compared between many different tissues. We have screened the output of RDA by microarray in order to rapidly confirm differential expression of RDA fragments derived from specific mRNA and to greatly increase the breadth of differential fragments cloned (17).

2. RDA

RDA is a method to detect DNA fragments present in one pool (tester) that are not in another (driver). Representative fragments from each population are first generated by restriction endonuclease digestion of DNAs followed by PCR amplification. The resulting mixtures are termed 'amplicons'. The amplicons are then subjected to successive rounds of subtractive cross-hybridization followed by differential PCR amplification. This leads to progressive enrichment of fragments that are present in the tester pool but not in the driver.

RDA was first described to clone unique fragments between two populations of genomic fragments (1), and has since been adapted to analysing differences between cDNA populations (4). The application of RDA to cDNA instead of genomic DNA created unique challenges. Though genomic RDA and cDNA RDA are similar, different determinants need to be taken into consideration in order for these procedures to be successful. In genomic RDA, the populations of fragments being compared are significantly more complex but most single copy sequences are present in comparable amounts. By comparison in cDNA RDA, the cDNA pools are much less complex, but there is large variability in cDNA (expression) levels from different genes.

To use RDA to detect differentially expressed genes, cDNAs (instead of genomic DNAs) are generated from two cell populations being compared. The RDA protocol consists of four steps:

- cDNA synthesis (*Protocol 1*)

- amplicon preparation (*Protocol 2*)

- subtractive hybridization (*Protocol 3*)

- differential PCR amplification (*Protocol 4*)

Repeating the third and fourth steps two to four times usually results in cDNA fragments that derive exclusively from differentially expressed transcripts. These fragments can then be subcloned and analysed further.

2.1 General considerations for RDA

A number of critical determinants have emerged from our experience with RDA. First, the relative difference in expression level impacts whether a gene is recovered by RDA. In a mixed population of differentially expressed genes in which some genes differ by fivefold and others by 100-fold, the genes whose expression differ by 100-fold will be amplified preferentially in RDA. However, absolute expression level has not been a crucial determinant for identifying genes because fragments from both abundant and rare transcripts have been isolated (5). Secondly, like all subtractive methods, RDA only allows comparison of two cell populations at a time. Thirdly, each RDA experiment only leads to the recovery of 6–12 differentially expressed cDNA fragments which likely represent only a small subset of all the differentially expressed genes (4–12). Finally, RDA has generally required large ($\sim 100 \, \mu g$) quantities of starting RNA which precludes using non-renewable cell sources such as tumour specimens.

The effect of preferentially enriching the highly differentially expressed genes is most pronounced if three or four cycles of RDA are performed rather than one or two cycles. In the end, there is a tradeoff between the relative enrichment for differentially expressed genes and the complexity of RDA output. If only a few (6–12) highly differentially expressed genes are sought with very low non-differentially expressed gene contamination, three or four cycles of RDA should be performed, and screening by microarray is not necessary as the products can be easily distinguished by gel electrophoresis and directly cloned. On the other hand, if larger populations of differentially expressed genes are desired, the RDA should be limited to one or two cycles of subtraction. Under these conditions, specific bands are difficult to detect in the smear of PCR fragments by gel electrophoresis. In this case, microarray screening is highly advantageous to screen out non-differentially expressed genes and select for a non-redundant set of differentially genes most efficiently (16, 17).

The fact that some cDNA fragments amplify better than others in the PCR reaction also has an effect on cRDA output. In order for a gene to be represented in RDA amplicon pools, it must have appropriate restriction sites positioned within it that upon digestion yield a fragment that amplifies efficiently. Considering this, it seems unlikely that a single restriction enzyme would suffice for all differentially expressed genes. In fact, it appears that any single RDA experiment detects only a subset of the genes that are differentially expressed. Consistent with this is the fact that different restriction enzymes used for amplicon preparation often alters the subset of differentially expressed genes detected in a given experiment. If an increased breadth of differentially expressed genes is desired, additional restriction enzymes should be used.

2.2 Practical considerations for RDA

RDA allows the pairwise comparison of any two cDNA populations (e.g. A and B). It is advisable that the two reciprocal comparisons are made in a given experiment (i.e. A – B and B – A subtractions are performed in parallel). Each serves as a good control for the other. If bands appear in one comparison that are not in the reciprocal comparison, there is a very high likelihood that they derive from differentially expressed genes.

The ideal number of subtractions required for a given set of comparisons may need to be determined empirically. Most of our successful experiments have been performed after two rounds of RDA subtraction when comparing similar tumour tissues. In tissues where there is a predominance of genes expressed at a low level, one additional round of subtraction may be required to reduce the number of non-differentially expressed genes to be screened by microarray.

Some technical considerations are notable. Volumes and temperatures are important. A micropipettor that is accurate to 0.1 μl is very helpful. Spin column technologies have been used frequently to circumvent extractions with phenol and chloroform. While spin columns from Qiagen, Inc. have been adequate, other similar devices could probably be used as well.

Protocol 1. RNA extraction and cDNA preparation from archived tissue specimens

Reagents

- STAT-60 lysis solution (Tel Test, Inc.)
- Oligo(dT) latex beads (Oligotex, Qiagen, Inc.)
- 5 × first strand buffer (Gibco BRL, Inc.)
- RNase inhibitor (10 U/μl) (Gibco BRL, Inc.)
- 0.1 M DTT
- dNTP mix: 5 mM final concentration of dATP, dCTP, dGTP, dTTP
- 0.5 μg/μl oligo(dT)$_{12-18}$ (Gibco BRL, Inc.)
- 10 μg/μl BSA

- Superscript II reverse transcriptase (200 U/μl) (Gibco BRL, Inc.)
- 5 × DS buffer: 100 mM Tris pH 7.5, 500 mM KCl, 30 mM MgCl$_2$, 50 mM (NH$_4$)$_2$SO$_4$, 250 μg/ml BSA
- 15 mM βNAD (Sigma)
- *E. coli* polymerase I (10 U/μl) (Gibco BRL, Inc.)
- RNase H (3 U/μl) (Gibco BRL, Inc.)
- *E. coli* ligase (10 U/μl) (Gibco BRL, Inc.)

Method

1. Cryostatically section 10–20 μm thick slices from fresh frozen tissue blocks.[a]

2. Place 20–30 sections into 1 ml STAT-60 or RNAzol lysis buffer and process according to manufacturer's recommendations.[b]

3. Quantitate RNA by absorbance at 260 nm and check RNA integrity by loading 1 μg on a formaldehyde agarose minigel.

4. Bind 30–100 μg total RNA to oligo(dT) latex beads according to manufacturer's recommendations.

5. Elute poly(A)$^+$ RNA from latex beads and reduce to 29 μl total volume by rotary vacuum apparatus.

6. Denature RNA by heating to 70 °C for 10 min and put on ice.

7. For first strand cDNA synthesis, add the following ingredients in order:
   - 10 μl 5 × first strand buffer
   - 0.5 μl 10 U/μl RNase inhibitor
   - 0.5 μl 0.1 M DTT
   - 5 μl 5 mM dNTP mix
   - 3 μl 0.5 μg/μl oligo(dT)$_{12-18}$
   - 0.5 μl 10 μg/μl BSA
   - 1.5 μl Superscript II reverse transcriptase[c]

8. Incubate at 37 °C for 1–2 h.

9. For second strand cDNA synthesis, place reaction on ice and add the following in order:
   - 25 μl dH$_2$O
   - 20 μl 5 × DS buffer

46

- 1 μl 15 mM βNAD
- 0.5 μl 0.1 mM DTT
- 2.5 μl 10 U/μl *E. coli* polymerase I
- 0.4 μl 3 U/μl RNase H
- 0.5 μl 10 U/μl *E. coli* ligase

10. Incubate at 16°C for 2–3 h.

11. Extract reaction mixture with 100 μl phenol:chloroform (1:1) and ethanol precipitate cDNA.

12. Resuspend cDNA pellet in 20 μl dH$_2$O and analyse 4 μl by agarose gel electrophoresis.[d]

---

[a] Archived fresh frozen tissues are usually stored as blocks suspended in OCT medium.
[b] The yield of RNA can vary widely with the size of the tissue block as well as the source and condition of the tissue prior to freezing.
[c] If starting with less than 50 μg total RNA, add 1 μl [^{32}P]dATP to act as tracer.
[d] It is important to confirm that the gel profiles of cDNA samples to be compared by RDA are nearly identical to each other.

Protocol 2. Generation of amplified cDNA fragments ('amplicons')

Equipment and reagents

- 10 × *Dpn*II buffer (New England Biolabs)
- *Dpn*II (10 U/μl) (New England Biolabs)
- 10 × ligase buffer (New England Biolabs)
- T4 DNA ligase (New England Biolabs)
- 10 × PCR buffer (pH 8.4, no Mg^{2+}) (Perkin Elmer–Cetus)
- dNTP mix: 2.5 mM final concentration of dATP, dCTP, dGTP, dTTP
- 25 mM MgCl$_2$
- RBgl24 oligo (2 μg/μl): 5'-AGCACTCTCCA-GCCTCTCACCGCA-3'
- RBgl12 oligo (1 μg/μl): 5'-GATCTGCGGTGA-3'
- *Taq* polymerase (5 U/μl) (Perkin Elmer–Cetus)
- Qiaquick spin columns (Qiagen, Inc.)

Method

1. Digest double-stranded cDNAs with *Dpn*II by mixing 8–16 μl cDNA with 10 μl 10 × *Dpn*II buffer, 2 μl *Dpn*II in 100 μl total volume for 1–2 h at 37°C.[a]

2. Extract reaction mixture with 100 μl phenol:chloroform (1:1), ethanol precipitate, and resuspend DNA pellet in 43 μl dH$_2$O.

3. Add 6 μl 10 × ligase buffer, 4 μl 2 μg/μl RBgl24 oligo, and 4 μl 1 μg/μl RBgl12 oligo.

4. Heat to 55°C for 1–2 min in a heating block and then allow the block to cool for 1 h at 10°C.

Protocol 2. *Continued*

5. Add 3 μl T4 DNA ligase and incubate at 16°C overnight.

6. Dilute ligation mixture to 100 μl total volume with dH_2O.

7. Set up a pilot PCR reaction in a 200 μl thin wall microcentrifuge tube by mixing the following on ice:
   - 1 μl cDNA ligation mixture
   - 10 μl 10 × PCR buffer
   - 16 μl 25 mM $MgCl_2$
   - 10 μl 2.5 mM dNTP mix
   - 0.5 μl 2 μg/μl RBgl24
   - 62 μl dH_2O
   - 0.5 μl *Taq* DNA polymerase

8. Place PCR reaction in thermocycler pre-heated to 72°C, incubate for 5 min, and follow with the programme—95°C for 1 min; 72°C for 3 min—for 32 cycles.

9. Starting at cycle 17, withdraw 10 μl aliquots from the PCR reaction every three cycles (i.e. cycle 17, 20, 23, 26, 29).

10. Analyse PCR products on 1.2% agarose 0.5 × TBE minigels. For each PCR reaction, determine the minimum number of cycles beyond which further amplification does not occur.[b]

11. Perform 12 PCR reactions set-up according to steps 7 and 8 and using the optimized number of PCR cycles. At the end of the PCR programme, perform an additional 10 min incubation at 72°C, then cool to 25°C.

12. Pool similar PCR reaction tubes, extract with an equal volume of phenol:chloroform (1:1), ethanol precipitate, and resuspend DNA pellet in 350 μl dH_2O.

13. Add 40 μl 10 × *Dpn*II buffer and 10 μl *Dpn*II, and incubate at 37°C for 2–3 h.

14. Purify amplicons using Qiaquick spin columns by loading 100 μl *Dpn*II reaction per column.

15. Quantitate amplicons by absorbance at 260 nm.[c]

[a] If starting with less than 50 μg total RNA, digest all of the cDNA generated in *Protocol 1*. If starting with more RNA, use half.
[b] Amplicons will appear as a smear ranging from 200–1500 bp.
[c] While OD_{260} provides a reasonable estimate, it frequently overestimates the actual yield of amplicons due to partial contamination from adapter oligonucleotides. Dyes that specifically detect double-stranded DNA such as Picogreen (Molecular Probes, Inc.), provide a more accurate assessment but require a fluorimeter.

Protocol 3.   Subtractive hybridization of amplicons

Reagents

- JBgl24 oligo (2 μg/μl): 5'-ACCGACGTCGAC-TATCCATGAACA-3'
- JBgl12 oligo (1 μg/μl): 5'-GATCTGTTCATG-3'
- EEP buffer: 30 mM EPPS pH 8 (Sigma), 3 mM EDTA, 12.5% PEG (Sigma)

- TE buffer: 10 mM Tris pH 7.5, 1 mM EDTA
- NBgl24 oligo (2 μg/μl): 5'-AGGCAACTGT-GCTATCCGAGGGAA-3'[a]
- NBgl12 oligo (1 μg/μl): 5'-GATCTTCCCTCG-3'[a]

Method

1. For each amplicon population, create tester populations by ligating JBgl adapters to 0.5 μg amplicons in a total volume of 60 μl according to *Protocol 2*, steps 3–6.[b]

2. Set up subtractive hybridization by mixing 20 μl (0.1 μg) JBgl tester amplicons with 100 μl (10 μg) driver amplicons (from *Protocol 2*).[c,d]

3. Extract with 120 μl phenol:chloroform (1:1) and then with 120 μl chloroform.

4. Precipitate DNA by adding 30 μl 10 M ammonium acetate and 300 μl ethanol, and spin for 10 min at 12 000 g in a microcentrifuge. Wash pellet with 70% ethanol and dry completely.

5. Resuspend in 4 μl EEP buffer and overlay with 40 μl mineral oil.

6. Heat to 95–6 °C for 4 min, spin briefly in a microcentrifuge, and add 1 μl 5 M NaCl.

7. Incubate at 67 °C for at least 21 h.

8. At the end of incubation, dilute with 95 μl TE buffer.

[a] These oligos are to be used if a second round of RDA is to be performed.
[b] RDA is a pairwise comparison between two cDNA populations (e.g. population A versus B) performed by subtracting a tester population with a molar excess of driver amplicons. In general it is good practice to perform both A – B and B – A comparisons at the same time.
[c] The initial tester to driver ratio is 1:100. If a second round of RDA is performed, this ratio decreases to 1:400–800.
[d] A good positive control is to set up a mock hybridization using the same amount of tester but tRNA instead of driver amplicons.

Protocol 4.   Enrichment of cDNA fragments from differentially expressed genes

Equipment and reagents

- 10 × PCR buffer (no Mg^{2+}) (Perkin Elmer–Cetus)
- 25 mM MgCl$_2$
- dNTP mix: 2.5 mM final concentration of dATP, dCTP, dGTP, dTTP
- JBgl24 oligo (2 μg/μl)

- NBgl24 oligo (2 μg/μl)[a]
- *Taq* polymerase (5 U/μl) (Perkin Elmer–Cetus)
- Qiaquick spin columns (Qiagen, Inc.)
- 10 × *Dpn*II buffer (New England Biolabs)
- *Dpn*II (10 U/μl) (New England Biolabs)

Protocol 4. *Continued*

Method

1. Set up PCR reaction No. 1 in a 200 μl thin wall microcentrifuge tube by mixing the following on ice:
   - 10 μl hybridization mixture from *Protocol 3*
   - 10 μl 10 × PCR buffer
   - 16 μl 25 mM MgCl$_2$
   - 10 μl 2.5 mM dNTP mix
   - 0.5 μl 2 μg/μl JBgl24
   - 53 μl dH$_2$O
   - 0.5 μl *Taq* polymerase[b]

2. Place PCR reaction in thermocycler pre-heated to 72 °C, incubate for 5 min, and follow with the programme—95 °C for 1 min; 72 °C for 3 min—for ten cycles.

3. Set up the second PCR reaction as in step 1 using 10 μl of product from PCR No. 1.

4. Place PCR reaction in thermocycler pre-heated to 72 °C, and follow with the programme—95 °C for 1 min; 72 °C for 3 min—for 24 cycles.

5. Starting at cycle 15, withdraw 10 μl aliquots from the PCR reaction every three cycles (i.e. cycle 15, 18, 21, 24).

6. As in *Protocol 2*, analyse PCR products on 1.2% agarose 0.5 × TBE minigels. For each PCR reaction, determine the minimum number of cycles beyond which further amplification does not occur.[c]

7. Repeat PCR No. 2 in quadruplicate (steps 2–3) using the optimized number of cycles and adding an additional 10 min incubation at 72 °C at the end before cooling to 25 °C.

8. Pool similar PCR reaction tubes, extract with an equal volume of phenol:chloroform (1:1), ethanol precipitate, and resuspend DNA pellet in 175 μl dH$_2$O.

9. Add 20 μl 10 × *Dpn*II buffer and 5 μl *Dpn*II, and incubate at 37 °C for 1 h.

10. Purify fragments using Qiaquick spin columns by loading 100 μl *Dpn*II reaction per column.

11. Pool and quantitate fragments by absorbance at 260 nm.

12. Subtracted fragments can be subcloned into plasmids for microarray analysis (see *Protocol 5*). Alternatively they can be ligated to NBgl

adaptors and subject to another round of RDA according to *Protocols 3* and *4*.

[a] This primer is used if a second round of RDA is being performed.
[b] Enrichment of cDNA fragments present in tester over driver is accomplished by a two step amplification process; an initial PCR reaction is followed by a dilution step and a final PCR amplification.
[c] After one round of subtraction, PCR products generally appear as a smear with a more narrow size range (200–1200 bp) than initial amplicons. After two rounds of subtraction, the size range decreases further and individual bands can usually be seen.

3. Generation of libraries from RDA subtractions

After shotgun ligation of the RDA products, which is generally efficient because four nucleotide overhangs can be used in the cloning, a mini-library is created in a bacterial host (*Protocol 5*). Pick only as many bacterial colonies as will be screened. The recombinant bacterial colonies are transferred directly into 96-well plates containing glycerol-based medium for growth and long-term storage (*Protocol 6*). This provides a convenient system for retrieving and distributing clones. After the bacterial colonies are grown to saturation, the 96-well plates can be frozen and maintained at –80°C for many months.

Individual inserts from each recombinant plasmid are amplified with vector-specific primers. The conditions in *Protocol 7* work well for amplification from pBluescript, as well as many other vectors. There is no need to purify individual plasmid DNAs for PCR amplification to generate sufficient insert for microarray preparation.

Protocol 5. Shotgun subcloning of RDA fragments

Equipment and reagents

- pBluescript vector (Stratagene)
- *Bam*HI endonuclease (New England Bio-labs)
- 10 × NEB *Bam*HI buffer (New England Bio-labs)
- Calf intestinal phosphatase (New England Biolabs)
- T4 DNA ligase (New England Biolabs)
- 10 × T4 DNA ligase buffer (New England Biolabs)
- Electrocompetent Top10 *E. coli* (Invitrogen)
- Selective agar Petri plates: LB with 1.5% agar, 100 μg/ml ampicillin, 0.1 mM IPTG, 25 μg/ml X-Gal

Method

1. pBluescript vector is prepared for shotgun cloning of the subtracted products. 10 μg supercoiled vector is cleaved in 1 × NEB *Bam*HI buffer with 40 U *Bam*HI in a final volume of 200 μl over 4 h at 37°C. 200 ng are electrophoresed on 1% agarose and ethidium bromide stained to assay digestion.

2. The digested vector is dephosphorylated by adding 12 U CIP to the digestion reaction and incubating at 37°C for 1 h. The DNA is recovered after phenol:chloroform extraction by ethanol precipitation.[a]

Protocol 5. *Continued*

3. 200 ng subtracted fragments from *Protocol 4* are mixed with 200 ng pBluescript from step 2 in 1 × ligation buffer and 400 U T4 DNA ligase, and incubated at 16°C for 12–18 h.

4. 45 μl ddH$_2$O is added to the ligation with 5 μg tRNA as carrier and ethanol precipitated, washed with 70% ethanol, air dried, and resuspended in 5 μl ddH$_2$O.

5. 1–5 μl ligation product is added to freshly thawed electrocompetent cells, mixed on ice, and electroporated with a Bio-Rad Gene Pulser set at 1.8 kV in 0.1 cm cuvettes.[b]

6. 1 ml SOC media pre-warmed to 37°C is added to the cuvette, the bacteria suspended and transferred to 5 ml culture tubes, and grown with moderate agitation on a rotary shaker at 37°C for 45 min.

7. Three dilutions of the transformed bacteria are plated onto selective agar plates. Dilution one is 100 μl transformed bacteria in SOC. Dilution two is 10 μl bacteria mixed with 90 μl LB. Dilution three is 1 μl bacteria mixed with 99 μl LB. Each dilution is applied to a separate selective agar plate and rubbed in with a sterile glass rod. The remainder of the bacteria in SOC are stored at 4°C.

8. Agar plates are incubated overnight at 37°C, placed in a refrigerator for several hours, and white recombinant colonies are identified.[c]

9. The dilution that yields a suitable density of recombinant plasmid-containing colonies (500/plate) is selected for further plating from the residual bacteria in SOC. Typically, libraries with 2000 independent recombinants are sufficient for near exhaustive screening of the RDA subtraction. The library is picked and gridded as in *Protocol 6*.

[a] If cloning efficiency is low, the efficiency of digestion of pBluescript and CIP treatment can be tested by ligating treated vector in the absence of insert. 100 ng ligated empty vector should yield fewer than 100 colonies.
[b] It is reasonable to test the efficiency of transformation of the electrocompetent cells with 1 ng supercoiled pBluescript plasmid. A transformation efficiency of 10^7 transformants/μg plasmid DNA is generally sufficient for this shotgun cloning.
[c] Prolonged incubation at 4°C enhances the blue colour and makes the recombinant colonies easier to identify.

Protocol 6.   Picking transformed libraries for long-term propagation

Equipment and reagents

- Sterile 96-well v-bottom culture plates (Costar)
- Growth media (LB): 100 μg/ml ampicillin, 7% glycerol

Method

1. Individual colonies are picked with a sterile toothpick or pipette tip and transferred into a single well of a 96-well culture plate containing 200 μl growth media. 96 clones are transferred into each plate. Typically, 10–12 96-well plates of clones are picked from each transformed RDA subtraction product library.

2. 96-well plates are incubated at 37 °C and grown for 14 h with gentle rotation until cultures appear cloudy.

3. The plates can now be stored at –80 °C for long-term storage of the arrayed library, or subjected to amplification of the cloned insert in 96-well plate format as described in *Protocol 7*.

4. Microarray fabrication

A variety of technologies are available for microarray fabrication, including several commercial systems. We have found the system described by the Brown Laboratory (Stanford University) to work well, and instructions for the fabrication of a printing robot are available in electronic form (`http://cmgm.stanford.edu/pbrown/mguide/index.html`). However, we incorporate some simpler means to attach PCR products to the glass slides which are detailed in *Protocol 7*. Slides that are coated with poly-L-lysine or modified covalently with amino-alkyl silane perform well for microarray fabrication. The slides should be inspected visually to exclude slides containing water spots or other visible surface defects. We routinely print microarrays in batches of 138 1″ × 3″ glass slides. The number of slides printed depends on the arrayer configuration used.

Protocol 7. Amplification of RDA inserts in 96-well plate format for arraying

Equipment and reagents

- MJ Research PTC-100 thermal cycler with heated lid
- 10 × PCR buffer: 100 mM Tris pH 9, 500 mM KCl, 15 mM MgCl₂, 0.1% Triton X
- dNTP mix: 2.5 mM final concentration dATP, dGTP, dCTP, dTTP

- Amplitaq DNA polymerase (Perkin Elmer)
- Amplification primers: m13 forward, m13 reverse (Operon)
- 96-well v-bottom thermal cycler plates (Costar)
- Silanized slides (Sigma)

Method

1. For each 96-well plate to be amplified, prepare 5 ml PCR mix on ice in a sterile trough containing 1 × PCR buffer, 1 μM each primer, 0.1 U/μl *Taq* DNA polymerase, and 200 μM dNTPs. Aliquot 50 μl PCR mix per

Protocol 7. *Continued*

well into a PCR plate on ice, and add 0.5 µl per well of saturated bacterial culture from the 96-well culture plates using an 8-channel pipetting device.

2. Thermal cycling consists of an initial denaturation of 5 min at 96°C, followed by 34 cycles of 55°C for 40 sec, 72°C for 120 sec, and 94°C for 40 sec, with a final extension of 5 min at 72°C.

3. 5 µl of each PCR reaction is chromatographed by electrophoresis in 1% agarose and visualized by staining with ethidium bromide. Most PCR amplification products are 300–700 bp in size, and correspond to approx. 2 µg total amplified insert.

4. The remaining 45 µl of the PCR reaction is precipitated in the 96-well plates by addition of 4.5 µl 3 M sodium acetate pH 5.2 and 100 µl pure ethanol. The 96-well plates are incubated at –70°C for 1 h and the DNA is pelleted by centrifugation at 3000 *g* for 60 min at 4°C in a swinging-bucket rotor.

5. The precipitated DNA is washed once with 70% ice-cold ethanol. The ethanol wash is then decanted by inverting the plate and the pelleted DNA is dried to completion by vacuum.

6. The DNA pellets are resuspended in 10–15 µl 350 mM sodium carbonate pH 9.

7. The plates are covered, heated to 95°C for 5 min, and cooled on ice prior to arraying.

8. Using a robotic transfer device,[a] the DNA is transferred from the 96-well plates onto 40–138 silanized glass slides. A four-pin transfer device will transfer DNA from 96-wells onto 138 glass slides in 40 min. Arraying should be performed in a dust-free environment. Once printed, the slides can be stored for months in a sealed container at room temperature.

[a] Various robotic devices for the transfer of small volumes of DNA solution onto glass slides have been described and some are commercially available. Our apparatus closely follows the original design developed by the Brown laboratory, which is available on the web (http://cmgm.stanford.edu/pbrown/array.html). Advanced printing technology is available commercially from Telechem (http://www.arrayit.com).

5. Microarray hybridization

Various hybridization conditions for microarrays have been published (13–15, 17). We have found that the strongest hybridization signals for RDA experiments are observed using hybridization *Protocol 8*. However, other hybridization conditions would probably also work well. The fluorescent nucleotides most frequently used are the Cy3 and Cy5 derivatives (Amersham). While there are some acceptable alternatives to Cy3 including avidin-phycoerythrin and 548 Alexa-dCTP (Molecular Probes), the simplest labelling conditions have been established using dCTP-Cy3 and dCTP-Cy5. These fluorescent nucleotide analogues allow direct incorporation into the DNA probe and still allow specific hybridization. In our experience, Klenow enzyme mediates the most efficient incorporation of these analogues into probes. While Cy3 is uniformly robust, the Cy5 signal can vary widely. In order to minimize variation, we recommend minimizing the number of freeze–thaw cycles of the stock solution and shielding the analogues from light at all times.

A number of devices have been fabricated to read the hybridized slides. We have fabricated a small desktop two-colour laser fluorimeter which scans the surface at 10 μm resolution, and scans up to a 25 × 50 mm area. The system is designed around a frequency doubled Nd-YAG laser (532 nm) and 635 nm diode laser. Details on the design are available on request. This device can be fabricated by APG, Inc. (`http://home.att.net/~apginc/fluor.htm`). Designs for other systems based on argon laser excitation are published on the web (`http://cmgm.stanford.edu/pbrown/scanner.html`). In addition, a desktop dual laser scanner (ScanArray 3000) is available from General Scanning with similar specifications. The fluorescence images can be analysed with *NIH-Image 1.61* on the Macintosh which allows convenient image analysis. For quantitation of each array element, we use *ImaGene 1.4* (BioDiscovery) which uses a deformable template to identify hybridized spots, performs signal analysis with local background subtraction, and exports the data into tab delimited spreadsheets.

Protocol 8.   Hybridization of cDNA amplicons to microarrays

Equipment and reagents

- Microarrays prepared using *Protocol 7*
- cDNA amplicons prepared using *Protocol 2*
- dCTP-Cy3, dCTP-Cy5 (1 mM stock) (Amersham)
- dNTP mix: 2.5 mM dATP, dTTP, dGTP, and 400 μM dCTP
- Klenow enzyme (New England Biolabs)
- 10 × Klenow buffer: 500 mM Tris pH 7.5, 100 mM MgCl₂, 10 mM DTT, 0.5 mg/ml BSA
- Random nonamers (6 mg/ml) (Operon)
- S200 Sephacryl spin columns (Pharmacia)
- Cot-1 DNA (1 μg/μl) (Gibco BRL)
- Ethanol

- 3 M sodium acetate pH 5.2
- Formamide (Fisher)
- 20 × SSC
- 10% SDS
- 50 × Denhardt's reagent: 10 mg/ml BSA, 10 mg/ml Ficoll 400, 10 mg/ml polyvinylpyrrolidone
- 60% dextran sulfate (Fisher)
- Stratalinker (Stratagene)
- Glass coverslips 22 × 22 mm (Fisher)
- Aluminium hybridization block
- Rubber cement

Method

1. Arrayed DNA slides are hydrated for 10–20 sec over a 37 °C water-bath and snap-dried on a metal block at 95 °C. The slides are then exposed to 400 mJ UV irradiation with a Stratalinker UV irradiator. The slides are

Protocol 8. *Continued*

then immersed in 0.1% SDS in water for 1 min, dH$_2$O at room temperature for 1 min, 95°C distilled water for 2 min, and 100% ethanol for 2
min. The slides are air dried and immediately ready for hybridization.[a]

2. Amplicons are labelled by random primer labelling. 2 μg of one of the
   two amplicons are mixed with 2 μl random nonamers, 5 μl 10 ×
   Klenow buffer, and dH$_2$O to a final volume of 43.5 μl. The mixture is
   incubated at 100°C for 3 min and transferred immediately to ice. 2 μl
   Klenow (10 U), 2.5 μl dNTP mix, and 2 μl dCTP-Cy3 are added in the
   dark, mixed, and incubated in the dark at 37°C for 12 h.[b] The same
   process is followed for Cy5 labelling of the second amplicon with
   substitution of dCTP-Cy5 for dCTP-Cy3.

3. Labelled samples are purified with S200 Sephacryl spin columns following the directions of the manufacturer. Blue (Cy5) or red (Cy3) colour
   should be easily visible in the labelled DNA which flows through the
   column. The labelled amplicons are mixed together with 5 μg Cot-1
   DNA and co-precipitated by the addition of 11 μl 3 M sodium acetate
   and 220 μl ethanol. After incubation at −70°C for 1 h, the sample is
   centrifuged at 14 000 *g* for 40 min, washed briefly with 70% ethanol,
   and air dried.

4. 15 μl hybridization buffer is added to the dried pellet. Final hybridization buffer is 50% formamide, 3 × SSC, 1% SDS, 5 × Denhardt's
   reagent, 5% dextran sulfate, made fresh weekly and stored at room
   temperature.

5. The sample is heated to 80°C for 10 min to denature the probe, cooled
   to 42°C, and hybridized to the microarray.

6. A 22 × 22 mm glass coverslip is placed carefully over the fluorescent
   sample to allow uniform sheeting of the probe over the entire DNA
   array. Care should be taken to avoid air bubbles.

7. The slide is placed on an aluminium block pre-warmed to 42°C and the
   edges of the coverslip sealed with rubber cement. The slide is then
   incubated at 42°C for 12–18 h.

8. The hybridized slides are washed in 2 × SSC plus 0.1% SDS for 2 min,
   0.2 × SSC for 2 min, and dH$_2$O for 30 sec. All washes are performed at
   room temperature. The slides are air dried to avoid water spots and
   scanned in a two colour laser scanning fluorimeter to quantitate fluorescent signal at each array element.

[a] Care should be taken not to allow spots to form on slides which will increase background. A
simple method for avoiding unwanted spots is to centrifuge the slides for 1 min at 500 *g* in a
swinging-plate rotor.
[b] The prolonged incubation for random primer labelling is necessary due to poor incorporation
of the nucleotide analogue by Klenow DNA polymerase.

6. Differential expression screening with microarrays

Microarrays of 400–1600 RDA products are typically sufficient to allow broad screening of the differentially expressed genes. Frequently, over 100 different products can be detected in a given experiment with a microarray containing 1600 elements. In general, two rounds of RDA subtraction yield a situation in which greater than 90% of the products arrayed are more abundant in tester than driver, and are thus detectable by microarray analysis. Clones that are not represented differentially are analysed in future hybridization experiments. The remaining clones are screened by repetitive probing of the microarray with mixtures of inserts from the arrayed library to create a non-redundant set of clones for DNA sequencing.

In a typical experiment, a set of 6–12 clones are generally representative of clones in the RDA library that would have been identified by further subtraction and gel analysis. It is advantageous to detect these clones early in the analysis. These clones frequently contribute the brightest hybridization signal in the differential hybridization of initial amplicons. Therefore, the 12 clones that have the strongest hybridization signals in probings with each amplicon are initially chosen for aggregate back-hybridization. Inserts from the 12 clones from each subtraction can be mixed and labelled as in *Protocol 7* and co-hybridized to the array as in *Protocol 8*. All positive hybridization signals are excluded from further analysis. Clones that did not hybridize are selected in batches of 12, mixed, labelled, and co-hybridized to the microarray until all clones have been analysed. An array of 1600 clones (800 from each direction of subtraction) can generally be screened in 20–40 back-hybridizations and will generate 100–200 difference products with minimal redundancy. In a typical printing of 138 slides, 20–40 are used for back-hybridizations leaving 100 slides for analysis of additional tissues and cell lines. Microarrays can be probed with labelled mRNA, cDNA, or amplicons. This allows a more thorough analysis of gene expression patterns in multiple tissues.

7. Summary

The protocols described in this chapter are primarily designed to expedite the analysis of gene expression from primary tissue specimens. Specific alterations of the original RDA protocol allow analysis of small amounts of biological material, thereby extending the application of RDA to biopsies and other minute specimens. The RDA process is typically limited to a few rounds of subtraction, which enriches for differentially expressed sequences and preserves the wide distribution of the differentially expressed genes. The complex molecular mixture from RDA is subcloned randomly into a plasmid vector, and the inserts are amplified and arrayed at high density at discrete positions onto glass slides. The arrayed inserts are subsequently co-hybridized with differentially labelled amplicons to identify those inserts that are differentially represented in the starting populations.

The merging of RDA and microarray analysis has proven to be an efficient method of detecting unique, differentially expressed genes. While we have focused on RDA, other subtractive techniques like SSH have also been screened by microarray hybridization in a similar format. Although the two techniques were not compared directly, a similar rate of unique differentially expressed genes were detected by SSH library screenings (L. Goodlick, J. Gregg, and S. Nelson, unpublished data).

The combination of RDA subtraction with microarray screening allows for a thorough analysis of differential gene expression between tissues. Because it is not currently practical to examine all gene expression patterns under all physiological conditions in a higher eukaryote, identifying subsets of cellular genes that are differentially expressed in particular disease states is one immediate benefit of coupling RDA and microarray technology. Coupling of RDA subtraction with microarray analysis creates a convenient, high throughput means by which to profile gene expression patterns.

References

1. Diatchenko, L., Lau, Y. F., Campbell, A. P., Chenchik, A., Moqadam, F., Huang, B., *et al.* (1996). *Proc. Natl. Acad. Sci. USA*, **93**, 6025.
2. Liang, P. and Pardee, A. B. (1992). *Science*, **257**, 967.
3. Lisitsyn, N., Lisitsyn, N., and Wigler, M. (1993). *Science*, **259**, 946.
4. Hubank, M. and Schatz, D. G. (1994). *Nucleic Acids Res.*, **22**, 5640.
5. Braun, B. S., Freiden, R., Lessnick, S. L., May, W. A., and Denny, C. T. (1995). *Mol. Cell. Biol.*, **15**, 4623.
6. Chu, C. C. and Paul, W. E. (1997). *Proc. Natl. Acad. Sci. USA*, **94**, 2507.
7. Dron, M. and Manuelidis, L. (1996). *J. Neurovirol.*, **2**, 240.
8. Edman, C. F., Prigent, S. A., Schipper, A., and Feramisco, J. R. (1997). *Biochem. J.*, **323**, 113.
9. Fu, X. and Kamps, M. P. (1997). *Mol.Cell. Biol.*, **17**, 1503.
10. Gress, T. M., Wallrapp, C., Frohme, M., Muller-Pillasch, F., Lacher, U., Friess, H., *et al.* (1997). *Genes Chromosome Cancer*, **19**, 97.
11. Lerner, A., Clayton, L. K., Mizoguchi, E., Ghendler, Y., van Ewijk, W., Koyasu, S., *et al.* (1996). *EMBO J.*, **15**, 5876.
12. Niwa, H., Harrison, L. C., DeAizpurua, H. J., and Cram, D. S. (1997). *Endocrinology*, **138**, 1419.
13. Schena, M., Shalon, D., Davis, R. W., and Brown, P. O. (1995). *Science*, **270**, 467.
14. Lockhart, D. J., Dong, H., Byrne, M. C., Follettie, M. T., Gallo, M. V., Chee, M. S., *et al.* (1996). *Nature Biotechnol.*, **14**, 1675.
15. DeRisi, J., Penland, L., Brown, P. O., Bittner, M. L., Meltzer, P. S., Ray, M., *et al.* (1996). *Nature Genet.*, **14**, 457.

16. Chang, D. D., Park, N. H., Denny, C. T., Nelson, S. F., and Pe, M. (1998). *Oncogene*, **16**, 1921.
17. Welford, S., Gregg, J., Chen, E., Garrison, D., Sorensen, P., Denny, C., *et al.* (1998). *Nucleic Acids Res.*, **26**, 3059.

4

Use of oligonucleotide arrays in enzymatic assays: assay optimization

STEPHEN CASE-GREEN, CLARE PRITCHARD, and
EDWIN M. SOUTHERN

1. Introduction

In the following chapter we show how assays commonly performed in solution and analysed by gel electrophoresis can be applied to solid supported oligo-nucleotides and oligonucleotide arrays (1). Primer extension (2) and ligation assays (3) for typing single nucleotide polymorphisms (SNPs) can be adapted to solid supports and modified for the analysis of short tandem repeats (STRs).

We should emphasize that none of the techniques described have been fully optimized for any individual target of interest; they rather provide a research tool to allow investigation of possible applications and to optimize specific assays involving oligonucleotide arrays. For instance, the methods of array synthesis we use are very convenient when a number of different systems are being used on a small scale (for research purposes), but other synthesis methods may be better if a large number of the same array is needed.

2. Fabrication of arrays

There are two general techniques for fabrication of oligonucleotide arrays. Either pre-synthesized oligonucleotides can be applied to the support, or *in situ* synthesis of oligonucleotides can be performed on the support. Both methods have advantages and disadvantages, some of which are summarized in *Table 1*.

In our laboratory we have developed methods based on *in situ* synthesis, using standard oligonucleotide synthesis reagents (4), which allow combin-atorial synthesis of multiple oligonucleotides in four steps (5). These 'barrier-based' methods are described in detail in the previous chapter. Different shaped masks to those for antisense scanning arrays are used in the following protocols (see *Figure 1*). Alternatively, pressing the support onto a block with

Table 1. Array manufacturing approaches

Manufacturing method	Deposition of pre-synthesized oligonucleotides	Synthesis of oligonucleotides *in situ*
Oligonucleotide synthesis	Serial	Combinatorial
Purification method	Standard methods usable	Purification not possible
Best method for	Many copies of the same array (production)	Single copies of different arrays (prototyping)

channels cut into it allows serial synthesis of oligonucleotides of unrelated sequence in a series of strips (6). If the oligonucleotides on an array are arranged in parallel lines, there is the opportunity to use it in more than one reaction if the samples to be hybridized are added in lines perpendicular to the oligonucleotides (7). Alternatively, the array can be cut into a number of strips for use in separate reactions (see *Figure 2*).

Assays described in this chapter are carried out on the functionalized polypropylene support described in the previous chapter (Beckman) (6, 8). This surface is suitable as a support for solid phase oligonucleotide synthesis. All syntheses in this chapter use 3'-dimethoxytrityl-5'-*N,N*'-diisopropylcyano-ethylphosphoramidites (reverse phosphoramidites). Deprotection leaves the oligonucleotides attached to the polypropylene via the initial, ammonia stable, phosphoramidate linkage to the 5' end of the oligonucleotide.

2.1 SNP array fabrication

The simplest type of array for polymorphism detection is prepared by the separate synthesis of each allele-specific oligonucleotide containing the variable

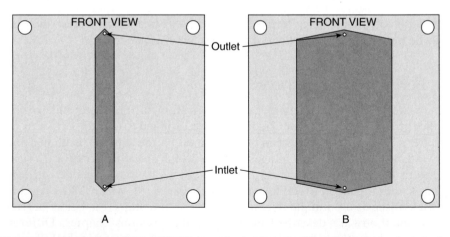

Figure 1. Layout of masks used for the synthesis of arrays. The dimensions given in the protocols refer to the width and height of the central rectangular region.

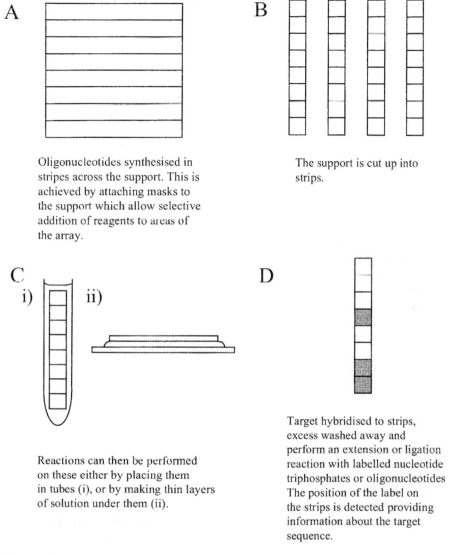

A

Oligonucleotides synthesised in stripes across the support. This is achieved by attaching masks to the support which allow selective addition of reagents to areas of the array.

B

The support is cut up into strips.

C

i) ii)

Reactions can then be performed on these either by placing them in tubes (i), or by making thin layers of solution under them (ii).

D

Target hybridised to strips, excess washed away and perform an extension or ligation reaction with labelled nucleotide triphosphates or oligonucleotides The position of the label on the strips is detected providing information about the target sequence.

Figure 2. Procedure for the analysis of DNA sequence via extension reactions involving immobilized oligonucleotides.

base at the terminal position distal to the support. This can be achieved in a number of different ways:

(a) A patch of the first oligonucleotide is synthesized on the support using a mask to direct the synthesis reagents. The mask is then moved to a position adjacent to the first oligonucleotide and the second oligonucleotide synthesized (*Protocol 1*). Use of a long thin mask (*Figure 1A*) minimizes reagent use and allows the array to be cut into strips in a perpendicular manner relative to the direction of array synthesis.

(b) A sequence that corresponds to the core sequence of the allelic oligo-nucleotides is synthesized. Then the mask is displaced by half a mask's width and a base corresponding to one of the alleles is added to the core sequence. A mask is then moved to the other half of the core patch, and the second allelic base is added.

Protocol 1. SNP array synthesis

Equipment and reagents

- DNA synthesizer (Perkin Elmer/ABI)
- Synthesis mask (*Figure 1A*)
- Glass or Perspex sheet
- Deoxynucleotide 3′-DMT, 5′-phosphor-amidites (Glen Research)
- Ammonium hydroxide solution

- Reagents for oligonucleotide synthesis (Perkin Elmer/ABI, Pharmacia, Cruachem)
- Duran bottle
- Aminated polypropylene support (Beck-man)
- Scalpel

Method

1. Clamp a mask (*Figure 1A*, 4 × 40 mm) to a piece of aminated poly-propylene using a G-clamp and a glass or Perspex backing plate.

2. Attach ports to the synthesizer and synthesize a patch of oligonucleo-tide corresponding to the first allele.

3. Displace the mask by 4 mm so that the mask is alongside the pre-viously synthesized patch.

4. Synthesize the oligonucleotide corresponding to the other allele.

5. Place the array in a Duran bottle, add 30% ammonia solution, seal the bottle securely, and heat at 55 °C for 6 h.

6. After allowing the bottle and contents to cool, remove the array, wash with ethanol, and dry. Store at –20 °C.

7. The array is cut into strips (1–2 mm wide) in a direction perpendicular to the strips of oligonucleotides using a scalpel.

2.2 STR array fabrication

The basic requirements for an array suitable for use in STR typing assay is shown in *Figure 3*. All the oligonucleotides of the array contain a sequence complementary to the region immediately adjacent to a repeat. This registration sequence forms a duplex between the target and the array oligonucleotides. The array oligonucleotides, each of which contain the flanking registration sequence, vary in the number of repeat units that they contain. Synthesis of

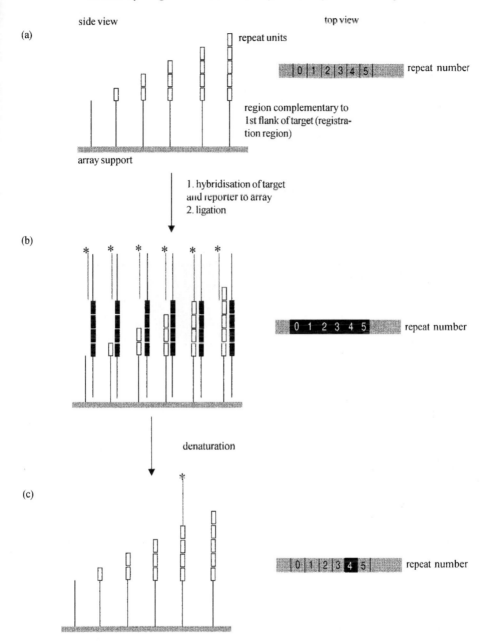

Figure 3. General scheme for the typing of short tandem repeats using enzyme ligase extensions to immobilized oligonucleotides. The addition of nucleotide triphosphates catalysed by polymerases can also be used in a similar manner.

Stephen Case-Green et al.

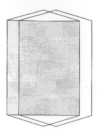

A patch of oligonucleo-
tide is synthesised on
the support containing
the registration sequence,
cctcccttatttcccctca and
five repeats,
ttcattcattcattcattca.

The mask is moved
by 5mm and a
sequence (ttca)
corresponding to one
repeat added.

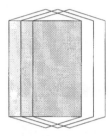
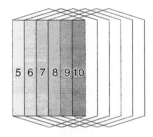

The mask is moved
by 5mm and a further
repeat added.

The moving of the mask
and synthesis of repeats
is continued a further
three times.

Figure 4. Synthesis of an array for the typing of the HUMTHO1 locus. The numbers on the lower right panel of the diagram represent the repeat lengths synthesized in these regions of the array.

these arrays can be carried out in a combinatorial manner using a variation on the methods described in the previous chapter for scanning array synthesis. *Figure 4* shows a scheme for the synthesis of an array for typing the HUMTHO1 locus.

Protocol 2. Short tandem repeat array synthesis

Equipment and reagents
• As for *Protocol 1*

Method

1. Clamp a mask (*Figure 1B*, 30 × 40 mm) to a piece of aminated poly-propylene using a G-clamp and a glass backing plate.

2. Attach ports to the synthesizer and synthesize a patch of oligonucleotide corresponding to the complement of the flanking sequence before the repeats of the target single-stranded DNA.

3. On top of this add a sequence complementary to the smallest number of repeats that may be present in the target DNA.

4. Displace the mask by 2 mm and synthesize a patch corresponding to one repeat.

5. Repeat step 4 until the maximum required number of repeats has been reached.

6. Place the array in a Duran bottle, add 30% ammonia solution, and heat at 55°C for 6 h.

7. After allowing the bottle and contents to cool, remove the array from bottle, wash with ethanol, and dry. Store at –20°C.

8. The array is cut into strips (1–2 mm wide) in a direction perpendicular to the strips of oligonucleotides.

3. Preparation of target DNA

To achieve efficient hybridization and enzymatic extension with the array oligonucleotides, a single-stranded DNA target (sample) is required. Since the DNA sample used for analysis is usually derived from a small amount of genomic material, an amplification method is normally needed. A two-step procedure can be used, whereby the sample is generated by PCR amplification followed by the digestion of the unwanted strand with an exonuclease (9). The primer used to amplify the strand of interest is synthesized such that the last five internucleotide linkages at the 5′ end contain phosphorothioate (10) linkages which protect the strand against exonuclease digestion. After PCR conditions are optimized, T7 gene 6 exonuclease is used digest the unwanted (unphosphorothioated) strand. The resulting single-stranded DNA sample can then be hybridized without further purification. Alternatively, standard purification techniques could be used.

Protocol 3. Preparation of single-stranded targets

Equipment and reagents

- PCR reagents
- PCR primer for the target strand containing 6 phosphorothioate linkages at the 5′-most 6 phosphate linkages
- Thermal cycler
- T7 gene 6 exonuclease (Amersham)
- PCR purification kit (optional, Qiagen)

Method

1. Carry out PCR under conditions that yield the desired product.

Protocol 3. *Continued*

2. Add T7 gene 6 exonuclease to give to a final concentration of 2 U/μl.

3. Incubate at 25°C for 1 h.

4. Incubate at 80°C for 5 min.

5. If desired, purification can be carried out using a commercially available purification kit.

4. Hybridization to arrays

The usefulness of oligonucleotide arrays is in their ability to bind to target nucleic acids in a sequence-specific manner, and allow unbound material to be washed away. In the simplest assay type, target sequences are distinguished by their ability to bind to complementary oligonucleotides on the array (6). This requires careful control of hybridization conditions so that different oligonucleotide/target interactions having different energies, produce different hybridization signals. When using hybridization in conjunction with enzymatic extension, the hybridization conditions can be less stringent because assay selectivity is enhanced by the enzyme.

Hybridization to oligonucleotides attached to solid supports is dependent on the same variables as hybridization in solution. Temperature, salt concentration, time, target concentration, and the addition of other reagents all affect hybridization signal. In the case of ligation reactions, the reporter oligonucleotide is added along with the target during the hybridization reaction.

Protocol 4. Hybridization

Equipment and reagents
- Buffer: 1 M NaCl
- Petri dish
- Tissues
- Forceps
- Strip of oligonucleotide array (30 mm × 2 mm)
- Target single-stranded nucleic acid

Method

1. Prepare a sample containing the target (1–5 pmol) in 100 μl buffer.

2. Soak a tissue in 1 × buffer and place around the inner perimeter of a Petri dish to create a chamber with 100% humidity.

3. Place the sample as a single 100 μl droplet in the middle of the Petri dish and place a strip of array (30 mm × 2 mm) on top.

4. Incubate for 1 h at the required hybridization temperature.

5. Remove the array from the hybridization solution and blot dry.

Protocol 5. Hybridization of target and reporter oligonucleotide to arrays

Equipment and reagents

- 1 M NaCl
- Petri dish
- Tissues
- Forceps
- Target single-stranded nucleic acid

- Labelled reporter oligonucleotide containing 5′ phosphate group
- Strip of oligonucleotide array (30 mm × 2 mm)

Method

1. Follow *Protocol 4*, except that the reporter oligonucleotide (5–10 pmol) is added to the hybridization mixture in step 1.

---

5. Enzyme catalysed extension reactions

5.1 Single nucleotide polymorphism (SNP) assays

There are many possible variants of the hybridization/extension method suitable for the analysis of (biallelic) single nucleotide polymorphisms (SNPs) (11, 12). In the simplest form, two oligonucleotides are synthesized that differ only in their terminal base, with one of the two oligonucleotides being perfectly complementary to the target to be analysed. Hybridization of the target sequence will occur with similar efficiency to both oligonucleotides due to the poor discrimination at terminal bases (13). Ligases and polymerases can however distinguish the two duplexes formed. These enzymes are able to carry out enzymatic extension only if a perfect duplex is present. *Table 2* summarizes

---

Table 2. Array assay summary

	Polymerase	Ligase
Reaction catalysed	Addition of a nucleotide to the 3′ end of a nucleic acid using deoxynucleotide triphosphate source.	The formation of a phosphate linkage between the 3′ hydroxyl and a 5′ phosphate. Addition of a deoxyoligonucleotide.
Oligonucleotide attachment to the solid support	5′ end attachment only, assay requires free 3′ hydroxyl.	5′ or 3′, but mismatch of a 3′ base likely to produce greater discrimination—5′ attachment may therefore be preferable.
Labelling procedure for nucleotide or oligonucleotide	Fluorescent, radioactive, biotin.	Fluorescent, radioactive, biotin.

---

relevant information for the use of ligases and polymerases in these assays. By adding DNA polymerase and a labelled nucleotide triphosphate complementary to the first base 5′ to the allelic position in the target, enzymatic extension will occur on array oligonucleotides that form perfect duplexes with the target. The spatial location of the label on the solid support indicates array elements that share the complementary sequence to the target (*Figure 5A*). In the ligation method, the labelled reporter oligonucleotide and the target are hybridized and ligated to the array (*Protocol 5*) (*Figure 6A*). In our hands, *Thermus thermophilus* DNA ligase is suitable for most assays (14), as it combines high purity with good discrimination and activity over a large temperature range (15).

In a variation that is applicable to both assays, the oligonucleotides on the array terminate at a position one base upstream of the base in the target to be analysed. In polymerase assays, a labelled nucleotide triphosphate complementary to one of the alleles in the target is incorporated only if the target sequence contains its complement. The result can be confirmed by carrying out the reaction in the presence of other bases that should give the opposite result (*Figure 5B*). Ligation can also be used in this assay, whereby the nucleotide triphosphates are substituted with labelled reporter oligonucleotides having terminal bases complementary to the alleles to be analysed (*Figure 6B*).

5.2 Short tandem repeat (STR) typing

A method for measuring STR length is shown in *Figure 2*. As with SNP typing, assays using DNA ligases and DNA polymerases are feasible. In the basic STR ligation assay, the target sequence and reporter oligonucleotide complementary to the distal flanking region to the repeat are hybridized to an array of oligonucleotides containing a guide registration sequence plus a varying number of repeats. The ligase can only join the labelled oligonucleotide with the oligonucleotide on the array when a perfect duplex junction is formed. Perfect duplex junctions only occur when the array contains oligonucleotide repeats with lengths equal to those of the target (16).

The polymerase method is similar to the ligase utilizing method. STRs in which the first base of the repeat unit is non-complementary to the first base following the repeat are analysed. Labelled nucleotide triphosphate complementary to the first base after the repeat are incubated on the array in the presence of DNA polymerase. The labelled nucleotide is incorporated only in cases where the repeat number on the array precisely matches that of the target. To confirm the assay results, the reaction can be repeated using a labelled nucleotide triphosphate complementary to the first base of the repeat. Only array oligonucleotides shorter than the target repeat size will extend in this case.

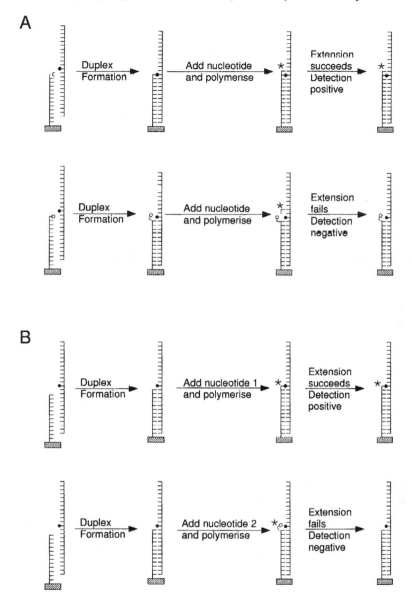

Figure 5. General scheme for typing single nucleotide polymorphisms (SNPs) using polymerase catalysed extensions on immobilized oligonucleotides. (A) Extension on allele-specific oligonucleotides with a nucleotide triphosphate. (B) Extension on a common oligonucleotide using allele-specific nucleotide triphosphates.

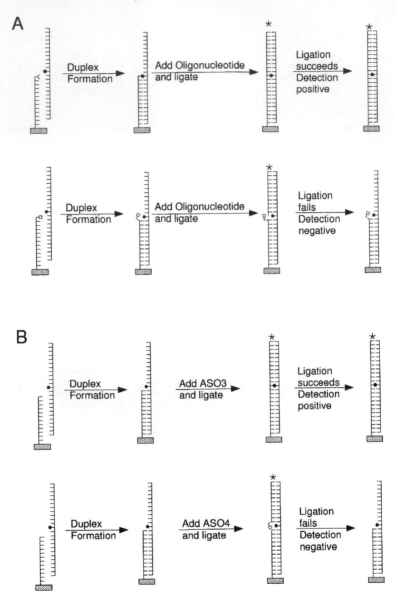

Figure 6. General scheme for the typing of single nucleotide polymorphisms using ligase catalysed extensions to immobilized oligonucleotides. (A) Ligation to allele-specific oligonucleotides with a common reporter. (B) Ligation to a common oligonucleotide using allele-specific reporters.

Protocol 6.   Ligation

Equipment and reagents

- 5 × ligation buffer: 100 mM Tris–HCl pH 8.3, 0.5% Triton X-100, 50 mM MgCl$_2$, 250 mM KCl, 5 mM NAD$^+$, 50 mM DTT, 5 mM EDTA
- Petri dish set up as humid chamber
- *Thermus thermophilus* DNA ligase (*Tth* DNA ligase) (Advanced Biotechnologies Ltd.)
- Forceps

Method

1. Prepare a solution of DNA ligase (1 U/μl) in 1 × ligase buffer and place as a single drop in a humidified Petri dish.
2. Add a strip of array (30 mm × 2 mm) hybridized according to *Protocol 5*.
3. Incubate at 37 °C (or 65 °C for STR arrays) for 1–8 h.
4. Heat water:formamide solution (1:1, v/v) at 100 °C for 5 min.
5. Blot dry and image.

Protocol 7.   Primer extension by polymerase

Equipment and reagents

- 5 × polymerase buffer: 200 mM Tris–HCl pH 7.5, 100 mM MgCl$_2$, 250 mM NaCl
- Polymerase dilution buffer
- 100 mM DTT
- T7 Sequenase V2. (13 U/μl) (Amersham)
- Humid chamber
- Dideoxynucleotide triphosphate: [^{33}P]ddNTP (450 μCi/ml) (Amersham)
- Forceps
- TE buffer: 10 mM Tris–HCl pH 8, 1 mM EDTA pH 8

Method

1. Prepare 40 μl of a solution containing Sequenase (0.5 U/μl), DTT (2.5 mM), polymerase buffer (1×), and the appropriate ddNTP (25 nCi/μl).
2. Soak a tissue in water and place round the inside of a Petri dish.
3. Add the solution as a puddle to the middle of the Petri dish.
4. Float a strip of pre-hybridized array (*Protocol 4*, 1 mm × 30 mm) on the solution.
5. Incubate at 37 °C for 1 h.
6. Wash away unbound material with TE buffer at 65 °C for 5 min.
7. Blot dry and image.

---

6. Variations on protocols

The following variations are regularly used in the protocols described.

6.1 Direction of oligonucleotide synthesis

Polymerase catalysed extension requires the oligonucleotides to be attached to the solid substrate through their 5′ ends. For ligation-based protocols, the oligonucleotides on the array can be attached by either the 5′ or 3′ end, using the methods described in *Protocols 1* and *2*. Either deoxynucleotide 5′-dimethoxytrityl-3′-phosphoramidites or the deoxynucleotide 3′-dimethoxytrityl-5′-phosphoramidites are used in the two scenarios. A requirement for ligation with oligonucleotides is that the 5′ end must contain a free phosphate group. This can be achieved by reacting the growing oligonucleotide chain with a chemical phosphorylating reagent such as a 'phosphate-on' phosphoramidite available from most DNA synthesis reagent suppliers. The phosphoryl-adding phosphoramidite is added at the last step in the chemical synthesis of the oligonucleotides. Free phosphate groups can also be added post-synthesis using polynucleotide kinase and ATP, a reaction that works either on oligonucleotides in solution and those tethered to solid substrates.

6.2 Linkers

The use of a chemical linker between the solid surface and the oligonucleotides provides advantages of improving the efficiency of hybridization and increasing access of the oligonucleotides to enzymes. Addition of chemical linkers based on polyethylene glycol (17) and deoxythymidine phosphoramidites (18) have both been used to add linkers prior to oligonucleotide synthesis.

6.3 Hybridization/reaction chamber

Performing hybridizations and other biochemical reactions with array strips in droplets allows the volume of liquid to be minimized; however, the chamber has to be made as humid as possible to prevent evaporation of the sample especially at elevated temperatures. The protocols above utilize Petri dishes containing wetted tissues, but wetted laboratory tissues can also be draped over the outside of the Petri dish. Alternatively, the Petri dishes can be placed in sealed plastic containers or sealed tubes. Although the sample volumes in reactions involving sealed containers or tubes are often greater than in droplets of solution, sealed vessels can be more easily incubated on hot blocks or in water-baths.

6.4 Hybridization buffers

The hybridization buffers can be varied from those described herein. Using a two-step process for the hybridization and enzymatic reaction procedures allows for different buffers to be used for the hybridization and enzymatic steps.

6.5 Hybridization temperature

Hybridization temperature can be varied in a manner analogous to the hybridization buffer. Many enzymes require specific temperatures, but by using a two-step hybridization/reaction procedure (or one-step methods, see below), the hybridization and enzymatic steps can be performed at different temperatures.

6.6 Labelling

Radiolabels were used in the protocols described here. Radioisotopes are convenient for many applications as they are readily available commercially and easily detected using a PhosphorImager. Other label types can also be used and, in most cases, these labels can be purchased as ready-to-use reagents. We have used Cy5 labelled oligonucleotides in ligation assays and Cy5-linked nucleotide triphosphates in polymerase extension assays. The Cy5 label can be detected using a STORM PhosphorImager. Due to the high background fluorescence of polypropylene when excited at short wavelengths, we have found that fluorescein is not compatible with polypropylene.

6.7 Nucleotide triphosphate

The extension method described in *Protocol 7* utilized dideoxynucleotide triphosphate (ddNTP). For most applications, the appropriate deoxynucleotide triphosphate (dNTP) can also be used.

6.8 Enzyme

The protocols above use *Thermus thermophilus* DNA ligase for ligation reactions and Sequenase for the extension reactions. Other enzyme types can also be used and have advantages if certain temperatures are required, particularly those involving 'all-in-one' reactions (see below). In these cases, *Taq* and Thermosequenase have both been used successfully.

6.9 'All-in-one' reactions

Instead of performing the assays in two steps, the hybridization and enzyme-based ligation or polymerization steps can be performed in a single reaction. 'All-in-one' reactions place additional constraints on the reaction conditions, as the majority of enzymes work in a restricted range of temperatures and salt concentrations. The single-stranded target DNA generally needs to be purified. There are several advantages to 'all-in-one' reactions, including speed and signal amplification arising from the ability to cycle the temperature, thereby allowing the target DNA to be used as a template for multiple ligation or polymerization reactions.

References

1. Case-Green, S. C., Mir, K. U., Pritchard, C. E., and Southern, E. M. (1998). *Curr. Opin. Chem. Biol.*, **2**, 404.
2. Landegren, U., Kaiser, R., and Hood, L. (1988). *Science*, **241**, 1077.
3. Suomalainen, A. and Syvanen, A. C. (1996). *Methods Mol. Biol.*, **65**, 73.
4. Brown, T. and Brown, D. J. S. (1991). In *Oligonucleotides and analogues: a practical approach* (ed. F. Eckstein), p. 1. IRL Press, Oxford, UK.
5. Southern, E. M., Case-Green, S. C., Elder, J. K., Johnson, M., Mir, K. U., Wang, L., *et al.* (1994). *Nucleic Acids Res.*, **22**, 1368.
6. Maskos, U. and Southern, E. M. (1993). *Nucleic Acids Res.*, **21**, 2269.
7. Matson, R. S., Rampal, J., Pentoney, S. L., Anderson, P. D., and Coassin, P. (1995). *Anal. Biochem.*, **224**, 110.
8. Matson, R. S., Rampal, B., and Coassin, P. J. (1994). *Anal. Biochem.*, **217**, 306.
9. Nikiforov, T. T., Rendle, R. B., Goelet, P., Rogers, Y.-H., Kotewics, M. L., Anderson, S., *et al.* (1994). *Nucleic Acids Res.*, **22**, 4167.
10. Zon, G. and Stec, W. J. (1991). In *Oligonucleotides and analogues: a practical approach* (ed. F. Eckstein), p. 87. IRL Press, Oxford, UK.
11. Schumaker, J. M., Metspalu, A., and Caskey, C. T. (1996). *Hum. Mutat.*, **7**, 346.
12. Pastigen, T., Kurg, A., Metspalu, A., Peltonen, L., and Syvanen, A. C. (1997). *Genome Res.*, **7**, 606.
13. Case-Green, S. C. and Southern, E. M. (1994). *Nucleic Acids Res.*, **22**, 131.
14. Barany, F. (1991). *Proc. Natl. Acad. Sci. USA*, **88**, 189.
15. Pritchard, C. E. and Southern, E. M. (1997). *Nucleic Acids Res.*, **25**, 3403.
16. Pritchard, C. E. and Southern, E. M. (1996). In *Innovation and perspectives in solid phase synthesis and combinatorial libraries* (ed. R. Epton), p. 499. Mayflower Scientific, Birmingham, England.
17. Shchepinov, M. S., Case-Green, S. C., and Southern, E. M. (1997). *Nucleic Acids Res.*, **25**, 1151.
18. Guo, Z., Guilfoyle, R. A., Thiel, A. J., Wang, R., and Smith, L. M. (1994). *Nucleic Acids Res.*, **22**, 5456.

5

Antisense oligonucleotide scanning arrays

JOHN K. ELDER, MARTIN JOHNSON, NATALIE MILNER,
KALIM U. MIR, MUHAMMAD SOHAIL, and EDWIN M. SOUTHERN

1. Introduction

Antisense oligonucleotides are short DNA sequences, typically between 15–25 nucleotides, that can bind to a complementary mRNA target by Watson–Crick base pairing and selectively inhibit the expression of the target gene from among the 80 000 or so estimated to be present in a typical mammalian cell (1, 2). This, in principle, makes possible the rational design of DNA-based therapeutic drugs for specific inhibition of any gene of known sequence. Antisense oligonucleotide drugs are currently in advanced stages of clinical trials for viral diseases and cancer (3, 4). Antisense oligonucleotides are also a useful tool in biological studies of gene function.

A major issue in antisense development is the selection of those reagents that work effectively. The ability to bind to the target mRNA influences the efficacy of an oligonucleotide as an antisense reagent. Oligonucleotides targeted to regions separated by only a few bases can have markedly different antisense effects (5). There is compelling evidence that the presence of secondary structure in mRNA influences the formation of intermolecular hetero-duplexes between the mRNA and the antisense oligonucleotide (5, 6). Computer programs such as *mfold* (7), designed to predict secondary structure of RNAs, have a limited utility in the selection of antisense oligonucleotides (5, 8); empirical selection of those reagents that can form stable hetero-duplexes with the target mRNA is more effective.

A robust method for selecting antisense reagents should have the potential to analyse all possible sites in the target in an automated fashion. Several methods have been developed that meet these criteria (8–11). Oligonucleotide scanning arrays (12) provide an excellent approach for achieving these goals. The combinatorial fabrication method reduces the number of synthesis steps needed to provide arrays for parallel, exhaustive analysis of all possible sequences in the target mRNA.

The scanning arrays comprise sets of oligonucleotides of various lengths, representing complements to the target mRNA. A series of oligonucleotides is made by coupling the bases to a solid surface in the order in which they occur in the complement of the target sequence. The reagents used for oligonucleotide synthesis are applied to a confined area on the surface of the solid support. If the mask used to retain the reagents were kept in the same place during all the synthesis cycles, the result would be a complete complement of the target sequence. If, however, the mask is shifted along the surface after each round of coupling, the result is a series of oligonucleotides, each one complementary to a region of the target sequence (see Section 2.3). This chapter describes the types of solid surfaces used to make arrays; the methods used to prepare synthesis masks and scanning arrays, hybridization reactions, and computer-aided analysis of the hybridization results.

2. Array fabrication

2.1 Substrate for making arrays

The choice of array substrate material and attachment chemistry are important considerations for making high quality arrays. A flat, impermeable surface is required for synthesis *in situ*. Glass has a number of favourable qualities. These include its wide availability, smooth surface, physical and chemical stability, transparency, and compatibility with radioactive and fluorescent samples. Polypropylene also has favourable physical and chemical properties. For the method of array fabrication described in this chapter, it is important to form a tight seal between the substrate material and the synthesis cell. Metals such as stainless steel or aluminium form tight seals with polypropylene. Teflon (PTFE) seals well against both glass and polypropylene. The surface must be stable to the reagents used in oligonucleotide synthesis. We use float glass (3 mm thick) or polypropylene (0.5 mm thick). Care must be taken not to damage the surface as scratches introduce high background. The attachment of the oligonucleotide to the surface must be stable. Terminal attachment with a spacer between the surface and oligonucleotide is desirable (13).

Aminated polypropylene prepared by plasma discharge in the presence of

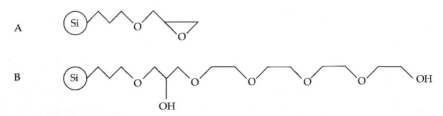

Figure 1. Chemical linkers. The first step in derivatization of glass (A) yields an epoxide group. The second step in derivatization (B) yields a hexaethylene glycol linker.

anhydrous ammonia was a gift of Beckman Instruments (Fullerton, USA), who have shown that oligonucleotide synthesis can proceed directly from amine groups on the surface of polypropylene (14). Silanol groups on the surface of glass are reacted with glycidoxypropyl trimethoxysilane to generate an epoxide group (*Figure 1A*). This is followed by reacting the epoxide group with a diol, leaving a linker terminating in a hydroxyl group from which conventional phosphoramidite chemistry can initiate (*Figure 1B*) (15).

Protocol 1. Derivatization of glass

Equipment and reagents

- Glass cylinder and apparatus as shown in *Figure 2*
- Water-bath at 80°C
- Glass sheets of required dimension (3 mm thick) (Pilkington, UK)
- 3 Glycidoxypropyl trimethoxysilane (98%) (Aldrich)
- Di-isopropylethylamine (99.5%) (Aldrich)
- Xylene (AnalaR) (Merck)
- Hexaethylene glycol (97%) (Aldrich)
- Sulfuric acid (AnalaR) (Merck)
- Ethanol (AnalaR) (Merck)
- Ether (AnalaR) (Merck)

Method

1. Prepare a mixture of glycidoxypropyl trimethyoxysilane, di-isopropyl-ethylamine, and xylene (17.8:1:69, by vol.) in a glass cylinder[a] (see *Figure 2*).

2. Place the glass plate(s)[b] in the mixture so that they are completely immersed and incubate at 80°C for 9 h.

3. Remove the plates from the mixture. Allow them to cool to room temperature and wash with ethanol and ether by squirting the liquid from a wash bottle.

4. Incubate the plates in hexaethylene glycol (neat) containing a catalytic amount of sulfuric acid (approx. 25 μl/litre) at 80°C for 10 h, with stirring.

5. Remove the plates. Allow them to cool to room temperature and wash with ethanol and ether.

6. Air dry the plates and store at –20°C.

[a] Final volume can be adjusted according to the size and number of plates to be derivatized.
[b] To keep the plates from touching, a 1–2 cm length of silicon tubing is cut and slit open. This is placed around the ends of the glass plates as illustrated in *Figure 2*.

2.2 Mounting polypropylene on glass

Unlike glass, polypropylene is not a rigid material and thus needs to be mounted on a solid, flat surface for its precise movement against the reaction mask during synthesis. We use soda glass (3 mm thick) for mounting poly-

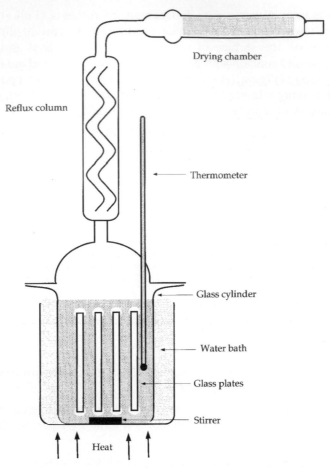

Figure 2. Apparatus for performing derivatization of glass plates.

propylene because it allows the flow of reagents through the reaction mask to be observed. Even mounting of polypropylene on glass is important to provide a good seal between the sealing edge of the reaction mask and the polypropylene surface—crucial to successful synthesis.

Protocol 2. Mounting polypropylene on glass

Equipment and reagents

- Soda glass sheet of the size of polypropylene[a]
- Polypropylene sheet cut to the correct size[b]
- Array maker (frame with mounted mask; see *Figure 5*)
- Knife or diamond scriber
- Photo Mount™ (3M)
- Ethanol
- Acetone

Method

1. Clean the glass sheet with ethanol and acetone and dry with forced air to remove dust particles.
2. Spray a very thin layer of Photo Mount on one side of the glass sheet.[c]
3. Place polypropylene on it taking care not to touch the reaction surface.
4. Cover the mount in cling film and place on a flat, clean surface, with polypropylene face down, under ~ 5–7 kg weight for 1 h.
5. Mark the first footprint of the mask on polypropylene by placing the mount in correct positions using a knife to create small notches in the polypropylene (*Figure 3*).[d]

[a] Glass used to mount polypropylene must be clean and free from dust particles because they can cause bulging of the polypropylene which can hinder the formation of a proper seal.
[b] The total area covered by an array for N bases using a mask of diagonal or diameter D and step size I mm is $N \times I + D$. 2–3 mm are added to margins to allow easy manipulations. For example, for an array made using a mask of 30 mm diagonal or diameter to cover a 100 nt sequence with 2 mm step size, a 234–236 mm long and 34–36 mm wide sheet is required.
[c] Avoid formation of lumps because they can create bulging of the polypropylene.
[d] After the synthesis is complete, also mark the last footprint of the mask. This helps registration of the template on the image for analysis (Section 2.8) and also allows the distance covered during synthesis to be checked. A diamond scriber can be used to mark glass.

2.3 Shapes and sizes of the masks

Both diamond-shaped and circular masks can be used to make scanning arrays. The maximum length of oligonucleotides synthesized depends upon

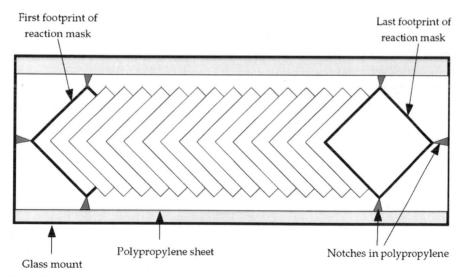

Figure 3. A completed array on polypropylene shown mounted on a glass support. The polypropylene has been notched to mark the first and the last footprints of the mask.

the ratio of the diagonal (for a diamond-shaped mask) or diameter (for a circular mask) of the mask to the displacement at each coupling step. For example, a diamond-shaped mask of 30 mm diagonal will produce 10-mers, 12-mers, or 15-mers using step sizes of 3 mm, 2.5 mm, or 2 mm, respectively. The smallest step size we have used is 1.5 mm with a 30 mm diamond-shaped mask. The length of the oligonucleotides is the number of bases that have been coupled at the point where the back of the mask passes the front. In this way it is possible to create arrays comprising sets of oligonucleotides of all sizes from monomers up to the longest in a single series of couplings by using a mask of appropriate size and shape. For example, a diamond-shaped template creates a series of small diamond-shaped cells (*Figure 4A*). The longest oligo-nucleotides are found at the centre and monomers are located at the edge. The cells created with a circular template differ in shape: along the centre line, they are lenticular, but off this line they form a four-cornered 'spearhead' that diminishes in size towards the edge (*Figure 4B*).

For each length of oligonucleotide s, there are $N - s + 1$ s-mers covering a total length of N bases. For example, if a 100 nt long sequence is covered in a 100 step synthesis, there will be 100 monomers and 86 15-mers. The last 14 positions in the sequence will be represented by shorter oligonucleotides only from 14-mer to monomer in this case. Therefore, for making 100 15-mers in an array, an additional 14 nt synthesis steps need to be added at the end (i.e. total coupling steps = $N + s - 1$).

The arrays as synthesized are symmetrical above and below the centre line of the template and each oligonucleotide is represented twice allowing for duplicate hybridization measurements (also see *Figures 4* and *8*).

2.4 Materials and machining of masks

Both diamond-shaped and circular reaction masks can be fabricated from stainless steel or aluminium: circular masks using a centre lathe and diamond-shaped masks using a horizontal milling machine. Circular masks can also be made from PTFE (Teflon). Diamond-shaped masks are more difficult to make with PTFE by the machining process but can be made by pressure moulding in a hydraulic press ($\sim$ 150 ton force) using a pre-machined die.

To make a diamond-shaped mask from metal (*Figure 5A*), the workpiece is held at an angle of 45° to the axis of the bed of the milling machine (the diag-onal of the diamond running parallel to the axis of the bed). The cavity is machined to the required depth (generally between 0.5–0.75 mm) to create a reaction chamber. The sealing edge (0.3–0.5 mm wide) is formed by machin-ing the outer lands to a depth of approximately 0.5 mm. The internal corners of the reaction chamber are radiused using the smallest possible diameter cut-ter ($\sim$ 1.5 mm). The sealing edge is finished by polishing flat with successively finer grades of wetted abrasive paper from $\sim$ P600 to P1200 (3M Inc. USA). The final polish is achieved by using a polishing grade crocus paper (J. G.

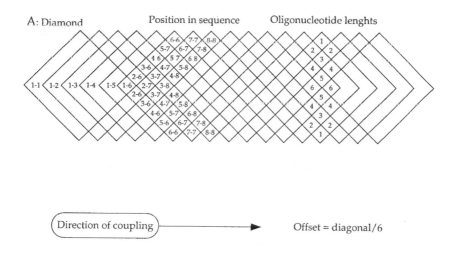

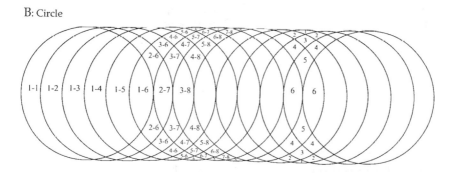

Figure 4. Organization of scanning arrays. Two template shapes are illustrated here, a diamond shape created by turning a square through 45° (A) and a circle (B). In either case, pressing a seal of the desired shape against the substrate on which the synthesis takes place creates a cell. Reagents, washing solutions, and gas are introduced at the bottom of the cell and removed from the top or the bottom. These processes can be carried out automatically by coupling the cell to an automatic DNA synthesizer such as the ABI 394. After each round of coupling, the cell is moved along the substrate by a predetermined step size. The longest oligonucleotides are made along the centre line and monomers are made at the edges. The arrays are thus symmetrical above and below the centre line allowing for duplicate measurement for each oligonucleotide. The length of the longest oligonucleotide is equal to the diagonal or diameter of the mask divided by the step size.

Naylor & Co Ltd., Woodley, Stockport, Manchester, England). Holes for reagent inlet and outlet are drilled, respectively, at the bottom and top of the reaction chamber (in the corners of the diamond) as close as reasonably possible to the sealing edge without damaging it. Care must be taken to de-burr

A

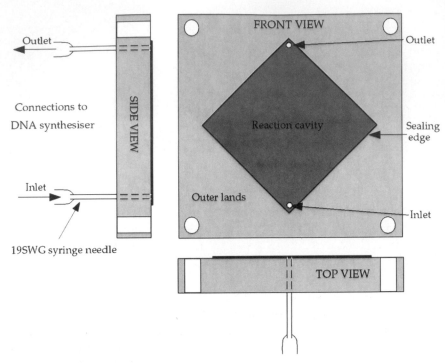

B

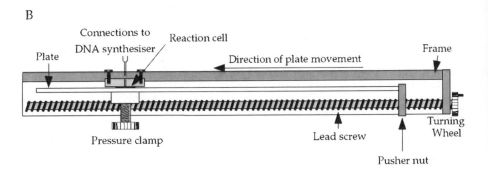

fully the holes at the point of entry into the reaction chamber. For PTFE masks the holes should be 1.0 mm diameter; for aluminium or stainless steel the holes should be 1.08 mm diameter. Inlet and outlet connections to the DNA synthesizer are made using standard 19SWG syringe needles (1.1 mm diameter) with the chamfered ends ground off and de-burred. They may be bent at ~ 45° at their midpoint to ease the space restriction when connecting up to the reagent lines of the DNA synthesizer. With PTFE masks, virtually

Figure 5. Apparatus used for applying reagents to the surface of glass or polypropylene. (A) A diamond-shaped metal mask. The mask consists of a 50 mm × 50 mm metal block with a diamond-shaped sealing edge, 0.5 mm height × 30 mm diagonal. Two holes of 1.08 mm diameter are drilled just inside the top and bottom corners of the diamond shape to take shortened 19SWG syringe needles used to connect the mask to the DNA synthesizer. The mask is fixed to the frame which carries the lead screw shown in (B). The inlet and outlet connections are fitted into the appropriate holes from the back by hand pressure only. (B) The apparatus is mounted on a frame made from 50 mm × 25 mm angle aluminium, fixed to the front of a DNA synthesizer. The lead screw, 1.0 mm pitch, is fitted with a pusher nut that drives the plate across the front of the mask. The driving wheel is marked in half-turns to enable the plate to be incremented forward in half-millimetre steps. The pressure clamp is a modified engineer's G-clamp fixed to the back of the frame with a polyethylene cushion mounted on its pressure pad. Moderate hand tightening is enough to seal the glass/polypropylene plate against the sealing edge of the mask.

100% leak-tight seal is obtained. In the case of aluminium or stainless steel masks, the 0.02 mm interference indicated above also provides a leak-tight seal without the use of any additional sealer. Care must be taken not to insert the end of the syringe needle into the reaction chamber void.

2.5 Making scanning arrays

The synthesis is carried out on an adapted ABI DNA synthesizer. The mask is fixed to the frame (*Figures 5B* and *6*) and its inlet and outlet are connected to the DNA synthesizer's reagent supply. The mask is sealed against derivatized glass or mounted polypropylene with a G-clamp. Sufficient pressure is applied to stop leakage but not enough to create indentations in the polypropylene surface which can lead to leakage of reagents from the mask during subsequent synthesis steps (approximately 500–800 Newton force). A slightly modified synthesis cycle is used (see *Table 1*). The flow times depend upon the size and the depth of the mask and have to be optimized for each mask. The cycles given in *Table 1* are typical for masks A and B.

Protocol 3. Making a scanning array

Equipment and reagents

- DNA synthesizer (ABI)
- Reaction mask and assembly frame
- Solid support (derivatized glass or polypropylene)
- Standard dA, dG, dC, and T CE phosphoramidites[a]
- Oxidizing agent[b]
- Acetonitrile
- Activator solution
- Deblock solution

Method

1. Program the DNA synthesizer with an appropriate synthesis cycle.

2. Enter the sequence in 5' to 3' direction.[c]

85

Protocol 3. *Continued*

3. Mark the first footprint of the mask on the polypropylene or derivatized glass surface by placing it in the desired starting position (Section 2.2).

4. Tighten the plate against the mask with the pressure clamp to produce a seal (*Figure 6*).

5. Start the DNA synthesizer to go through the pre-programmed cycle to couple the appropriate nucleotide.[d]

6. After completion of the step during the interrupt, slacken the pressure clamp and move the plate one increment.

7. Tighten the pressure clamp and start the synthesizer for the next nucleotide in the sequence. Continue the process until the full sequence length is synthesized.

[a] With the use of standard phosphoramidites in synthesis, the oligonucleotides are attached to the solid support at their 3' ends. Reverse phosphoramidites (Glen Research) can be used to make oligonucleotides that are attached to the solid support at their 5' ends.
[b] Iodine is used as an oxidizing agent to produce phosphodiester bonds between nucleotides. This can be replaced with a sulfurizing agent (Beaucage reagent, Cruachem) to make arrays of phosphorothioate oligonucleotides.
[c] The first condensation on the substrate is of the base at the 3' end of the sequence.
[d] At the start of each synthesis cycle, an 'interrupt step' can be introduced to halt the process at the first step for the next nucleotide condensation cycle to allow the operator to move the plate and restart the program.

It is difficult to monitor the efficiency of synthesis from the trityl yield due to the large amounts of the reagents used in coupling. However, several criteria suggest that the stepwise yield must be high. First, the ratio of coupling reagents to substrate is more than 200-fold greater in this format than in a conventional solid phase synthesis on a CPG column. For 1 nmol syntheses, we use quantities that would normally be used to make 0.2 mmol of the product. Secondly, the synthesis of any oligonucleotide on the array is dependent on successful coupling of each nucleotide. For example, each nucleotide residue in a 20-mer will occur in 19 other 20-mers. Thus successful synthesis of any one oligonucleotide, indicated by a positive hybridization signal, will indicate successful synthesis in these others. Although we cannot be sure that every coupling step has worked efficiently, synthesis of oligonucleotides using a cleavable linker and analysis by gel electrophoresis has suggested efficient yields (S. C. Case-Green, unpublished data).

2.6 Array deprotection

When using the standard nucleotide phosphoramidites, the exocyclic amines of the bases are protected chemically to prevent side reactions from occurring during synthesis; the protecting groups need to be removed from the coupled bases prior to hybridization.

Table 1. Program for the ABI394 DNA/RNA synthesizer to deliver reagents for one coupling cycle[a]

Step number	Function number	Function name	Step time A[b]	B[c]
1	106	Begin		
2	103	Wait	999	999
3	64	18 to waste	5	5
4	42	18 to column	25	60
5	2	Reverse flush	8	10
6	1	Block flush	5	5
7	101	Phos prep	3	3
8	111	Block vent	2	2
9	58	Tet to waste	1.7	1.7
10	34	Tet to column	1	3
11	33	B + tet to column	3	5
12	34	Tet to column	1	3
13	33	B + tet to column	3	5
14	34	Tet to column	1	3
15	33	B + tet to column	3	5
16	34	Tet to column	1	3
17	103	Wait	75	75
18	64	18 to waste	5	5
19	2	Reverse flush	10	10
20	1	Block flush	5	5
21	42	18 to column	15	40
22	2	Reverse flush	10	10
23	63	15 to waste	5	5
24	41	15 to column	15	50
25	64	18 to waste	5	5
26	1	Block flush	5	5
27	103	Wait	20	20
28	2	Reverse flush	10	15
29	1	Block flush	5	5
30	64	18 to waste	5	5
31	42	18 to column	15	35
32	2	Reverse flush	9	10
33	42	18 to column	15	35
34	2	Reverse flush	9	10
35	42	18 to column	15	35
36	2	Reverse flush	9	10
37	42	18 to column	15	35
38	2	Reverse flush	9	10
39	1	Block flush	3	3
40	62	14 to waste	5	5
41	40	14 to column	30	60
42	103	Wait	20	20
43	1	Block flush	5	5
44	64	18 to waste	5	5
45	42	18 to column	25	35
46	2	Reverse flush	9	10
47	1	Block flush	3	3
48	107	End		

[a] An interrupt is set at step 1 of the next base to allow the operator to move the plate one increment and restart the program. A long wait step at the beginning of the program is optional and is introduced if the operator does not wish to use the interrupt step. The operator is also advised to consult the user's manual for the DNA synthesizer.
[b] Step time for a diamond-shaped reaction chamber with 30 mm diagonal and 0.73 mm depth.
[c] Step time for a diamond-shaped reaction chamber with 54 mm diagonal and 0.51 mm depth.

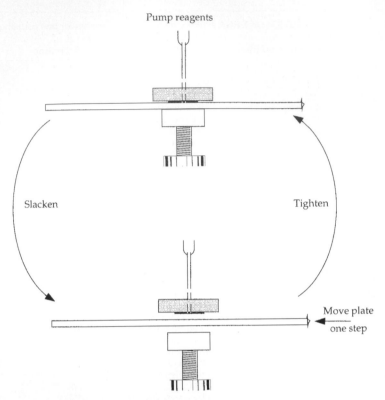

Figure 6. One coupling cycle comprises clamping the plate up to the mask, starting the DNA synthesizer to go through the pre-programmed cycle to couple the appropriate nucleotide, slackening the clamp, and moving the plate one increment by driving the lead screw the required number of whole or half-turns.

Protocol 4. Array deprotection

Equipment and reagents
- 30% ammonia solution (AnalaR) (Merck)
- High density polyethylene (HDPE) chamber (see *Figure 7*)
- Aluminium alloy plate
- 4 mm thick silicone rubber gasket
- Stainless steel M8 nuts and bolts
- Water-bath

Method
1. Place the glass or polypropylene[a] array(s) into the HDPE chamber.[b]
2. Add 30% ammonia into the chamber to cover the array(s) completely.
3. Place the silicone rubber gasket around the rim of the chamber.
4. Place the aluminium plate on top of the gasket.
5. Place bolts through the top plate, the rubber gasket and the HDPE chamber, and tighten.

6. Place the bomb in a water bath at 55°C for 12–18 h in a fume-hood.

7. Cool the bomb to 4°C before opening. The array is ready for use.

[a] Detach the polypropylene sheet from the glass mount by careful peeling from one end. The Photo Mount can be removed with acetone or ethanol.

[b] Polypropylene arrays can also be deprotected in tightly-sealed jam jars or Duran bottles.

Cross section

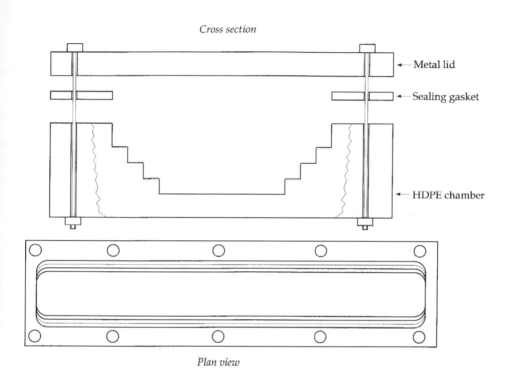

Plan view

Figure 7. Illustration of assembly for constructing deprotection bomb (not to scale).

2.7 Hybridization of a radiolabelled target to a scanning array

2.7.1 Preparation of radiolabelled target

An internally labelled RNA is used as a target to hybridize to a scanning array. The labelled product is generated by *in vitro* transcription in the presence of [α-^{32}P]UTP or [α-^{33}P]UTP (or [α-^{32}P]CTP) using an appropriate DNA template. *In vitro* transcription is generally carried out using T7 or SP6 RNA polymerase. A plasmid containing the desired DNA fragment under the transcriptional control of a T7 or SP6 promoter (such as pGEM; Promega) can be used as a template. The plasmid is linearized with an appropriate restriction endonuclease to produce transcripts of defined length without contaminating

Table 2. Bacteriophage promoter and leader sequences

Phage	Promoter/leader sequence[a]
T7	5' taa tac gac tca cta ta *ggg cga*
	5' taa tac gac tca cta ta *ggg aga*
SP6	5' att tag gtg aca cta ta *gaa tac*

[a] The hexanucleotide leader sequence (italics) appears in the transcripts.

vector sequence. If the required DNA fragment has not been cloned into such a plasmid, then a template for use with T7 or SP6 promoter can also be generated using the polymerase chain reaction. In the PCR-based scheme, primers are used to amplify the required fragment from a plasmid or genomic DNA, such that one of the primers has a T7 or an SP6 promoter/leader sequence added at the 5' end (*Table 2*).

Protocol 5. *In vitro* transcription using T7 or SP6 RNA polymerase

Reagents

- DNA template (at 0.5–1 μg/μl)
- T7 or SP6 RNA polymerase (Promega)
- Transcription buffer (5 × transcription buffer from Promega): 200 mM Tris–HCl pH 7.9, 30 mM $MgCl_2$, 10 mM spermidine, 50 mM NaCl
- RNase inhibitor (recombinant RNasin®; Promega)
- 100 mM DTT (Promega)
- [α-^{32}P]UTP (3000 Ci/mmol) or [α-^{33}P]UTP (2500 Ci/mmol) (Amersham)
- rNTPs (Pharmacia): ATP, GTP, and CTP stored as 10 mM solutions, and UTP as 250 mM in nuclease-free distilled water (Promega)

Method

The reaction below is for 20 μl using labelled UTP.

1. Add the following components to a microcentrifuge tube at room temperature in this order:

• 5 × transcription buffer	4 μl
• 100 mM DTT	2 μl
• RNasin®	20 U
• 10 mM ATP, GTP, and CTP	1 μl each
• 250 μM UTP	1 μl
• Template DNA	2 μl
• [α-^{32}P]UTP or [α-^{33}P]UTP	2 μl
• T7 or SP6 RNA polymerase	20 U
• Total volume	20 μl

2. Mix and incubate at 37°C for 1 h.

3. Remove 1 μl for quantitation (see *Protocol 6*).

4. Remove unincorporated label by Sephadex® G25 or G50 column chromatography.[a]

5. Save 1 μl of the purified transcript for quantitation in a microcentrifuge tube.

6. Check the integrity of the transcript by electrophoresis on a poly-acrylamide or agarose gel as described in Sambrook *et al.* (16).

[a] Ready-to-use columns are available from several suppliers including Promega and Pharmacia. Alternatively, spin columns made in-house, as described in Sambrook *et al.* (16), can also be used.

Protocol 6. Quantitation of transcripts

Equipment and reagents

- Scintillation counter (e.g. Beckman LS 1701)
- Scintillation vials
- Scintillation fluid (Amersham)

Method

1. Add 10 μl of the scintillation fluid to the samples saved in *Protocol 5*, steps 3 and 5.

2. Mix by vortexing and count the samples after placing the micro-centrifuge tubes in scintillation vials for 1 min.

3. Calculate the per cent incorporation:

$$\% \text{ incorporation} = \frac{\text{incorporated c.p.m.}}{\text{total c.p.m.}} \times 100$$

4. Calculate the amount of RNA synthesized:

$$\text{nmol } [\alpha\text{-}^{32}\text{P}]\text{UTP} = \frac{20 \ \mu\text{Ci}}{3000 \ \mu\text{Ci/nmol}} = 6.6 \times 10^{-3} \text{ nmol}$$

nmol cold UTP $= 1 \ \mu\text{l} \times 250 \ \mu\text{M} = 0.25$ nmol.

Total UTP $= 6.6 \times 10^{-3} + 0.25 = 0.256$ nmol.

For a reaction with 50% incorporation, the amount of UTP incorporated = 0.128 nmol.

Considering equal incorporation of all four nucleotides, total nucleotides incorporated

$$= 0.128 \times 4 = 0.512 \text{ nmol.}$$

Amount of full-length transcript = 0.512/total length of transcript.

Protocol 6. *Continued*

5. Calculate specific activity as below:

Total c.p.m. incorporated =

$$\text{incorporated c.p.m.} \times \text{dilution factor} \times \frac{\text{reaction volume}}{\text{volume counted}}$$

$$\text{Specific activity of RNA} = \frac{\text{total c.p.m. incorporated}}{\text{amount of transcript made}}$$

2.7.2 Hybridization

Scanning arrays made on glass are typically hybridized in a slightly different fashion from polypropylene arrays. For glass arrays, the hybridization solution is contained as a thin film of liquid between the array and a glass plate of the same size (*Protocol 7*). Polypropylene arrays are hybridized in a rotating tube placed in an oven (Techne) (*Protocol 8*).

An alternative method (*Protocol 9*) can be used with either a glass array or a polypropylene array attached to a flat backing plate. The hybridization solution is applied between the glass plate bearing the array and another plate of the same size. Three sides of the plate are sealed by inserting a single piece of silicone rubber cut into a 'U' shape between the plates.

Protocol 7. Hybridization to an array made on glass

Equipment and reagents

- Scanning array
- Hybridization solution: 1 M NaCl, 10 mM Tris–HCl, 1 mM EDTA, 0.01% SDS
- 50–100 fmol radiolabelled transcript (see *Protocols 5* and *6*)
- A glass plate of the same size as the array plate
- A moist chamber (a large plastic or glass lidded box containing wetted paper towels)
- Incubator
- Storage phosphor screen (Fuji or Kodak)
- PhosphorImager or STORM (Molecular Dynamics)

Method

1. Clean the glass plate (non-array) with acetone and ethanol and siliconize it by treatment with dimethyl dichlorosilane solution (Merck) and place in lidded hybridization chamber.

2. Place moist towel papers into the lidded box.

3. Dilute the radiolabelled transcript in an appropriate volume of the hybridization buffer (for an array of 250 mm × 50 mm use 500 μl).

4. Place items 1–3, the scanning array, and enough hybridization buffer to wash the array into the hybridization chamber in the incubator set at desired temperature (4–37 °C). Incubate for 30 min.

5. Pipette the hybridization mix (from step 3) in a line evenly along the length of the non-array plate such that no air bubbles form.

6. Starting at one end, carefully lay the scanning array plate face down on top of the hybridization mix. The mix will spread out and form a thin film of liquid between the scanning array and the non-array plate.

7. Hybridize for 3–4 h.

8. Separate the two plates from each other and wash the array plate with hybridization buffer to remove the unbound hybridization mix.[a]

9. Drain the plate and allow to air dry.[b]

10. Cover with cling film and expose on a storage phosphor screen for 16–20 h.

11. Scan the screen on a PhosphorImager and analyse the image using *xvseq* (Section 2.8).[c]

[a] The hybridization intensity is not affected by a longer wash time.
[b] For hybridizations below 37 °C, care must be taken not to touch the plates because this can lead to melting of short duplexes. For hybridizations below room temperature, the cling film and PhosphorImager screen must be cooled to the hybridization temperature and exposed at the same temperature.
[c] Use the smallest pixel size (50 μm on the STORM) to achieve the greatest accuracy for analysis. For a diamond array with a displacement of 2.5 mm this gives 50 pixels per width of each cell. An image generated from an array of 115 bases, with a mask size of 42.5 mm and displacement of 2.5 mm generates a file of around 15 megabytes.

Protocol 8. Hybridization to an array made on polypropylene

Equipment and reagents
- Hybridization solution: 1 M NaCl, 10 mM Tris–HCl, 1 mM EDTA, 0.01% SDS
- 50–100 fmol radiolabelled transcript (see *Protocols 5* and *6*)
- Hybridization tube and oven (Techne)
- Storage phosphor screen (Fuji or Kodak)
- PhosphorImager or STORM (Molecular Dynamics)

Method

1. Place the polypropylene array in the hybridization tube, coiling it in a spiral to ensure that the back of the array is touching the tube along its whole length, and such that the edges meet at each turn.

2. Dilute the radiolabelled transcript in an appropriate volume of hybridization buffer.[a]

3. Place items 1 and 2 in the oven at the desired temperature for 30 min.

4. Put 100 ml of washing buffer in the oven to equilibrate.

5. Pour the hybridization mix into the tube and hybridize for 3–4 h.

6. Pour off the hybridization mix and wash the array with the hybridization buffer.

Protocol 8. *Continued*

7. Allow the array to air dry, cover with cling film, and expose to a storage phosphor screen for 16–20 h (also see footnote to *Protocol 7*).

8. Scan the screen on PhosphorImager and analyse the image using *xvseq* (Section 2.8).

---

a Adjust the volume according to the size of hybridization tube. The mix should cover the array along the length of the tube. We use a 20 ml volume in a Techne hybridization tube.

Protocol 9. Alternative method for hybridization to glass or polypropylene arrays

Equipment
- A piece of silicone rubber (0.5 mm thick) cut into a 'U' shape to seal the plates
- Binder clips
- Syringe and needle

Method

1. Assemble the array and the non-array glass plate by inserting the silicone rubber between them and clamping them together with binder clips.

2. Dilute the radiolabelled transcript in the appropriate volume of hybridization buffer (5–10 ml).

3. Follow *Protocol 7*, step 4.

4. Apply the hybridization mix to the space between the two plates using a needle and syringe.

5. Make sure the array is horizontal.

6. Follow *Protocol 7*, step 7 onwards.

2.8 Computer-aided image analysis of scanning arrays

Visual inspection of a scanning array image will reveal the results generally, but computer-aided image analysis is needed to obtain quantitative information about hybridization intensities and the oligonucleotide sequences that generated them. We have developed a software package called *xvseq* to analyse scanning array images. A Sun Solaris binary version of the software is available by anonymous ftp (`ftp://bioch.ox.ac.uk/pub/xvseq.tar.gz`).

The program reads and displays images generated by a Molecular Dynamics PhosphorImager and can perform standard image manipulation operations such as scaling, clipping, rotation, and colourmap control. Its main purpose however is to calculate and display integrated intensities of array oligonucleotides, each of which corresponds to an image cell formed by the intersection of overlapping array templates. The user can specify the template size, shape, and location, step size between successive templates, as well as the sequence that generated the array pattern. The program superimposes the template grid on the array image, and the template parameters can be adjusted interactively so that the grid can be registered correctly with the hybridization pattern. Accurate registration is essential, especially for the circular template where cells shrink in size towards the upper and lower edges of the array, resulting in cells some of which may contain only a few pixels.

It can be difficult to achieve precise registration by reference to the hybridization pattern alone. Avoid placing the template grid so that it appears to be registered but is in fact misaligned by one or more template steps. This can occur when the hybridization signals at either edge of the array are weak or undetectable. Registration can be aided by the use of fixed reference points on an array such as those mentioned in Section 2.2.

Protocol 10. Stripping an array

Equipment and reagents
- Geiger-Müller counter (Mini-Instruments Ltd.)
- Microwave oven
- Storage phosphor screen (Fuji or Kodak)
- Magnetic stirrer
- PhosphorImager or STORM (Molecular Dynamics)
- Glass beaker, 500 ml
- Stripping solution: 100 mM sodium carbonate/bicarbonate pH 9.8–10, 0.01% SDS

Method

1. Heat the stripping solution in a microwave oven to 90°C in a glass beaker.

2. Immerse the array into the hot stripping solution and stir for 1–2 min with a magnetic stirrer.

3. Remove the array and wash it thoroughly with nuclease-free water, 70% ethanol, and finally with absolute ethanol.

4. Air dry the array.

5. Monitor with a Geiger counter to confirm that most of the radiolabel has been removed.[a]

6. Expose to a storage phosphor screen for 16–20 h and analyse on a PhosphorImager to verify complete removal of the radiolabel. The array is now ready for reuse.

[a] Repeat steps 1–4 if radioactivity on the surface of the array is still detectable.

After the template is registered, the program integrates cell intensities, normalized with respect to the number of pixels in each cell, allowing intensities

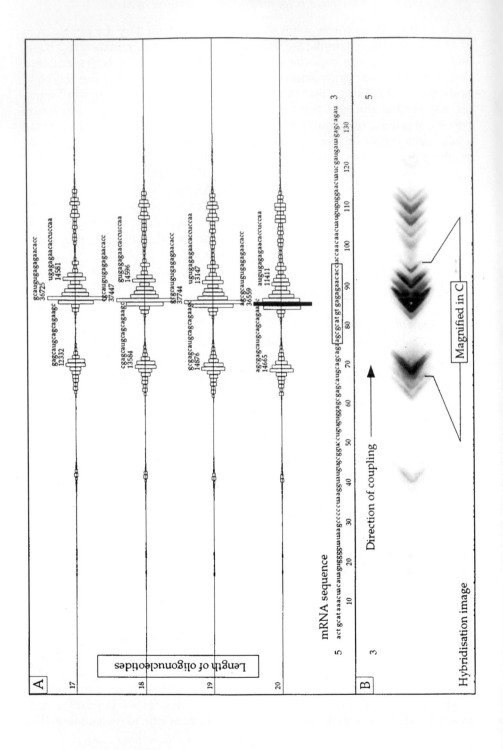

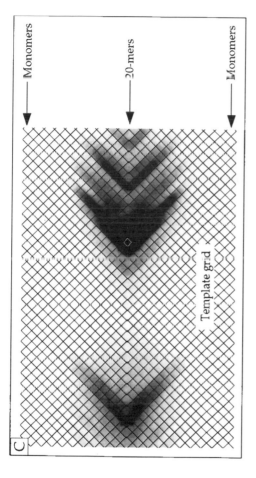

Figure 8. Display and analysis of results using *xvseq*. (A) The results of the integrated pixel values are displayed as paired histograms and the two values are for the areas above and below the centre line. Only values for 17-mers to 20-mers are displayed here but the program can display all values from monomers to the longest length of the oligonucleotides on an array. The program also includes tools to aid the interpretation of the large amounts of data in the figure. For example, clicking on a cell in the array highlights the corresponding region in the sequence (displayed under the histograms), the relevant bar in the histogram, and the integrated pixel values of the two cells. Clicking on a bar in the histogram (filled bar) highlights the corresponding cell of the array and the region in the sequence (boxed sequence). The values are of hybridization intensities of oligonucleotides on a single array and should not be used directly as comparators between different arrays. (B) Hybridization of a ^{32}P-labelled mRNA to an array of complementary antisense oligonucleotides. The array was made using a 30 mm diamond-shaped mask and a 1.5 mm step size on polypropylene. The longest oligonucleotides thus obtained were 20-mers found in a row of cells running along the centre line. The synthesis was in 3′ to 5′ direction. The sequence of the region of mRNA complementary to the array (the 'sense sequence') is written to a text file and is loaded before starting the integration process. A template grid comprising a series of overlapping diamonds, corresponding in number to the sequence length is placed over the image to generate cells containing individual oligonucleotide sequences. (C) A part of the image magnified with a template grid overlay. The smaller diamond shapes in the template grid correspond to individual oligonucleotide sequences. Each cell region is integrated.

of different cells to be compared directly. Pixels close to the cell borders are ignored when performing cell integrations. This helps avoid inaccurate cell intensities due to minor template mis-registration or signal 'bleeding' from adjacent cells.

The results can be displayed graphically in a variety of formats, including histograms of hybridization intensities along an entire sequence, or histograms of all oligonucleotide hybridization intensities centred about a particular point in the sequence. The results of a hybridization and their analysis using *xvseq* are shown in *Figure 8*.

2.9 Stripping of an array

The arrays can be reused several times. The radiolabelled target is removed from the array according to *Protocol 10*.

Acknowledgements

The authors wish to thank L. Wang, S. C. Case-Green, J. Williams, U. Maskos, and L. Baudouin for their assistance in the development of methods described in this chapter.

References

1. Antequera, F. and Bird, A. (1993). *Proc. Natl. Acad. Sci. USA*, **90**, 11995.
2. Fields, C., Adams, M. D., White, O., and Venter, J. C. (1994). *Nature Genet.*, **7**, 345.
3. Nyce, J. W. and Metzger, W. J. (1997). *Nature*, **385**, 721.
4. Webb, A., Cunningham, D., Cotter, F., Clarke, P. A., di Stefano, F., Ross, P., *et al.* (1997). *Lancet*, **349**, 1137.
5. Milner, N., Mir, K. U., and Southern, E. M. (1997). *Nature Biotechnol.*, **15**, 537.
6. Wagner, R. W., Matteucci, M. D., Grant, D., Huang, T., and Froehler, B. C. (1996). *Nature Biotechnol.*, **14**, 840.
7. Zuker, M. (1989). *Science*, **244**, 48.
8. Ho, S. P., Bao, Y., Lesher, T., Melhotra, R., Ma, L. Y., Fluharty, S. J., *et al.* (1998). *Nature Biotechnol.*, **16**, 59.
9. Lima, W. F., Brown-Driver, V., Fox, M., Hanecak, R., and Bruice, T. W. (1997). *J. Biol. Chem.*, **272**, 626.
10. Ho, S. P., Britton, D. H. O., Stone, B. A., Behrens, D. L., Leffet, L. M., Hobbs, F. W., *et al.* (1996). *Nucleic Acids Res.*, **24**, 1901.
11. Chen, T.-Z., Lin, S.-B., Wu, J.-C., Choo, K.-B., and Au, L.-C. (1996). *J. Biochem.*, **119**, 252.
12. Southern, E. M., Case-Green, S. C., Elder, J. K., Johnson, M., Mir, K. U., Wang, L., *et al.* (1994). *Nucleic Acids Res.*, **22**, 1368.
13. Shchepinov, M. S., Case-Green, S. C., and Southern, E. M. (1997). *Nucleic Acids Res.*, **25**, 1155.

14. Matson, R. S., Rampal, J. B., and Coassin, P. J. (1994). *Anal. Biochem.*, **217**, 306.
15. Maskos, U. and Southern, E. M. (1992). *Nucleic Acids Res.*, **20**, 1679.
16. Sambrook, I., Fritsch, E. F., and Maniatis, T. (ed.) (1989). *Molecular cloning: a laboratory manual*, 2nd edn. Cold Spring Harbor Laboratory Press, NY.

6

Application of ink-jet printing technology to the manufacture of molecular arrays

THOMAS P. THERIAULT, SCOTT C. WINDER, and
RONALD C. GAMBLE

1. Introduction

Massively parallel assay technology is increasingly the method of choice for conducting scientific inquiry in the physical sciences. For example, in physics, particularly materials science, combinatorial mixtures of components are prepared and screened to elucidate new superconductors. In chemistry, combinatorial synthesis programs represent one state-of-the-art mode for the discovery of novel drug leads. And in biology, arrays of unique DNA sequences are commonly used to assay the genetic state of cells. What these three different pursuits share is the need to perform a very large number of tests to achieve a particular goal. In all cases, small volumes of liquids must be precisely metered at high rates of speed. Technology derived from the ink-jet printing industry has been applied to meet such liquid handling needs.

This article focuses on the use of ink-jet technology for the manufacture of DNA microarrays. There are basically two modes of DNA microarray fabrication using ink-jets. First, there is the step-by-step synthesis of DNA by applying reactive nucleotide monomers to individual surface sites (1). Secondly, there is the spotting and immobilization of pre-synthesized DNA (2). Each technique has its particular advantages and disadvantages. As demonstrated below, the ink-jet approach can be applied successfully to either method of array fabrication.

2. Ink-jet technology

Ink-jet technology has been used for over 20 years to control delivery of small volumes of liquid to defined locations on two-dimensional surfaces. *Table 1* lists several modes of droplet generation. Common methods used in the consumer printer market combine a static pressure ink reservoir, a small

Table 1. Ink-jet methods

Device	Description	Notes
Piezoelectric capillary	Capillary with defined orifice, piezo generates pressure pulse.	Diameters of 25 μm readily achieved, up to 10 kHz.
Piezoelectric cavity	Micromachined structure and orifice with piezo pressure transducer.	Smaller diameter droplets and higher frequency than piezo capillary.
Thermal	Micromachined structure and orifice with thermal pressure transducer.	Smaller diameter droplets and higher frequency than piezo capillary.
Acoustic	Focused sonic pressure causes ejection of droplets from liquid surface.	No nozzle. High rates of drop formation (5 mHz) small drop diameters (1 μm).
Continuous flow	Stream of liquid broken into distinct droplets by oscillatory pressure. Droplets selected by charge or magnetism.	Robust system once started.

diameter orifice, and a pressure generating element. The orifice plays a significant role in determining the diameter of the droplets ejected from the device. Important goals of this mode of printing are to retain the ability to generate drops on demand and efficient ink consumption.

Another common mode of printing utilizes a continuous stream of droplets directed via an electric or magnetic field onto a print area or alternatively into a gutter where the ink is recycled. This printing mode is quite robust, as the jet is primed by pressurizing the liquid reservoir.

Finally, over the years, several intriguing technologies have been developed to generate droplets of liquid from reservoirs. One particularly interesting mode from the standpoint of biochemical applications is the nozzleless acoustic jet.

2.1 Piezoelectric capillary jets

One of the early jet designs was a glass capillary, fixed with an orifice, and surrounded by a cylindrical piezoelectric (3–5). A schematic of such a device is shown in *Figure 1*. Droplet formation with piezo capillary jets is accomplished by alternately expanding and contracting the piezoelectric element to generate shock pulses in the fluid chamber. When appropriately tuned to the characteristics of the liquid, pressure pulses sufficient to eject droplets from the nozzle can be generated. The typical rates of drop formation with these devices vary from single shot to approximately 10 kHz. Droplet formation is much easier at certain frequencies which are characteristic of the particular physical parameters of the jet device and liquid contained therein. The size of droplets from these devices depends upon the diameter of nozzle, the magnitude of the driving force, and the physical properties of the liquid in use. Appropriate care is required in manufacturing high quality nozzles and in

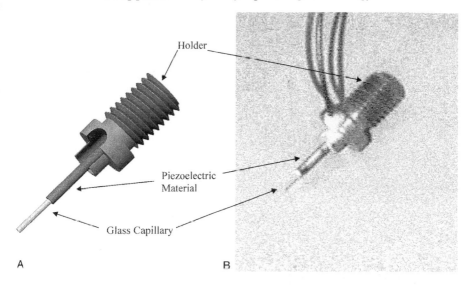

Figure 1. Piezoelectric capillary jet. (A) Device schematic (without leads or epoxy). (B) Typical jet.

supplying the correct waveform in order to obtain droplets that are satellite free and propagating perpendicular to the nozzle plate. A stroboscopic view of a droplet is shown in *Figure 2* along with a typical voltage waveform.

This very simple jet design has great flexibility in a variety of printing situations. Since only the glass capillary is brought into contact with the liquid reagent, these jets are compatible with a variety of chemical and biological applications. The physical dimensions of the device allow it to be used to directly sip load from microtitre well plates. Alternatively, tubing can be supplied to load the jet from the distal end, opposite the nozzle. One disadvantage of these devices is the relatively large amount of material that is required for loads in order to generate reproducible droplets. Typically, the volumes range from two to four microlitres. A sufficient amount of liquid must be used to fill the capillary from the nozzle to a point beyond the piezoelectric. Because of this limitation, these jets are most applicable when a large number of spots of the same material can be deposited.

A potentially interesting mode of printing with these devices was observed when the separation between the nozzle of the jet and the target surface was decreased to approximately one nozzle diameter. In this mode, the normal drop break-off does not occur. Instead, the extruding liquid from the nozzle contacts the surface and a much smaller than normal droplet of liquid is deposited. Presumably, the stoppage of forward momentum of the extruding droplet and the arrival of a low pressure front at the nozzle combine to bring the balance of liquid back into the jet. The diameter of the smaller droplet is

103

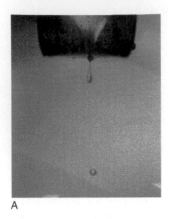
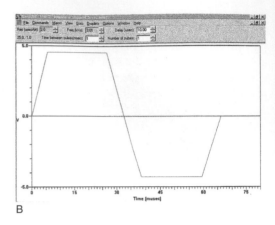

A   B

Figure 2. (A) Stroboscopic view of a steam of droplets. The droplets are being generated at a rate of ~ 6.5 kHz and are illuminated by a strobe light fired for 1.5 μsec intervals at the same frequency. The diameter of the droplet visualized is 30 μm and has a volume of approx. 33 picolitres. (B) Screen capture of waveform editor. A typical waveform used to generate droplets. Generally the slew rate for rise and fall is on the order of 10 V/μsec. The duration and magnitude of the pulse is tailored to the particular jet and the liquid to be jetted. Vertical scale is 10 V increments, horizontal scale is μsec increments. Window size is approx. 50 V by 80 μsec.

approximately the same as the nozzle diameter. Although this mode of printing could produce very small precisely placed droplets of liquid, it is quite difficult to control. The surface-to-jet separation is critical and must be maintained within a few microns. Further, the volume between the nozzle surface and the substrate can easily be filled by capillary action.

The piezo capillary jet device was used in the fabrication of two instruments:

(a) CombiJet, a molecular array synthesis device.

(b) GeneJet, a printing device for DNA microarrays.

Both of these instruments are discussed further below.

2.2 Other approaches

Each of the other devices in *Table 1* has its own set of advantages and limitations. The micromachined piezo or thermal jets (6, 7) could be used very effectively in molecular array construction. Precisely sized droplets can be generated due to the highly defined orifice geometry. In principle, these devices can be manufactured to very effectively use sub-microlitre volumes of liquid reagents to deliver droplets with diameters of ten microns or less. The main obstacle to the use of these devices is the specialized technology needed for their manufacture. Commercially available low cost devices are not configured in the most appropriate format for handling biological or chemical samples. This is due to very different goals in printing. Ink-jet printers are designed to maximize the rate of delivery of only a small number of different inks, typically four in the case of colour printing. Compatibility of components with the reagents used for chemical synthesis of arrays can be a concern. For constructing DNA arrays by deposition of gene fragments, the problem is to deliver tens of thousands of different reagents through the jet orifice. Additionally, unlike the piezo capillary jets, these micromachined devices typically cannot load directly from a microtitre well plate.

The continuous flow jet is also difficult to apply to the spotting of biological samples. Although its design allows for very robust droplet generation, it requires a relatively large volume of reagent as generally only a fraction of droplets that are generated are selected onto the printing surface. Most of the liquid must be recycled back in to the reservoir for effective use. At present this does not seem practical for molecular arrays due to the extremely small volumes of the liquid that carry the biological samples. Further, specialized modification would be required to handle large numbers of different samples.

Next under consideration are nozzleless acoustic jets which offer a unique method for drop generation (8–10). An acoustic beam is focused on the free surface of a liquid. Localized regions of high pressure cause droplets to be ejected from the surface. The size of the droplets depends on the sonic frequency and lens system. No nozzle is required to restrict the size of droplets that are expelled. However, the problem of passing many different samples through these jets will require some development. In the end, it could be extremely worthwhile, as the opportunity to generate exceptionally small droplets without fear of clogging a nozzle would be unique to this mode of jet.

In summary, the piezo capillary jets currently offer the best all round solution for drop generation for chemical and biological applications. As we shall see in the next section, these jets can be configured to deliver reagents required for oligonucleotide synthesis by combining a small number of jets together in a single synthesis instrument. A very similar instrument can be used where loading of biological reagents from microtitre plate wells is used to pass large numbers of samples through one or a smaller number of jets. At present, other types of jets can be configured for chemical synthesis provided the components are compatible with the solvents, etc., used in synthesis. However, without specialized instrumentation for loading samples, it will be difficult to use such jets in biological applications.

3. Molecular array fabrication by synthesis

In this section, instrumentation will be described that could be applied to a wide variety of molecular microarray fabrication applications. To date, instrument development has focused on using the piezoelectric capillary jets for making DNA microarrays. The first instrument, CombiJet, enabled synthesis

of DNA microarrays by delivering reagents for phosphoramidite oligonucleotide synthesis to defined locations on glass substrates. Two versions of
this instrument, one with a single jet and one with five jets, will be described.
The second instrument, GeneJet (described in Section 4), enabled the manufacture of DNA microarrays by spotting pre-synthesized DNA fragments that
were supplied in microtitre plate format.

3.1 *In situ* DNA synthesis

The use of ink-jet technology to deliver reagents takes advantage of the liquid
handling capability of the technology. Reagents can be used very economic-
ally as they are only delivered to the defined locations on the two-dimensional
array where they are required. It is possible to achieve localized DNA synthesis
by using jets to deliver reagents for one of two reactions in the phosphoramidite oligonucleotide synthesis cycle as shown in *Figure 3*. The first uses this
single jet device to deliver reagent to deprotect the 5′ hydroxyl position at
specific regions on the two-dimensional surface. In this mode, oxidation of the
phosphor and coupling of one of the four bases is done in a bulk chemical
treatment of the entire surface. The second method uses five jets, one for each
of the four phosphoramidites and one for the activating reagent. In this mode,
oxidation of the phosphor and removal of the 5′ protecting group are done in
a bulk chemical treatment.

3.2 CombiJet synthesizers

The CombiJet series of instruments were designed to allow for automated
oligonucleotide synthesis on glass microscope slides. The first instrument was
designed to be placed inside a nitrogen filled glove box. It contained a single
jet that was filled with a reagent for removal of the 5′ *O*-dimethoxytrityl protecting group. After selective deprotection, an operator manually moved the
microscope slide through the base coupling and oxidation reaction baths. The
second generation instrument, CombiJet II, provided a set of five jets used to
carry the four phosphoramidite bases and tetrazole. On this instrument, automated base coupling would occur. The operator would then move the slide
through the bath style chambers to perform the oxidation and 5′ OH deprotection. These research prototype instruments were used for proof of principle. Knowledge was acquired on how to modify the phosphoramidites
synthesis to make it compatible with ink-jet delivery of reagents.

CombiJet III was designed to fully automate all steps of DNA microarray
synthesis. A device schematic and photograph are shown in *Figure 4*. Like
CombiJet II, this instrument is capable of handling multiple jets. In its first
implementation, it operates in the single jet mode. A microscope slide is held
in a horizontal position in close proximity to an ink-jet device that was positioned to fire vertically upward. The jet is connected to a column that can hold
up to three millilitres of liquid reagent. Automated routines are used to con-

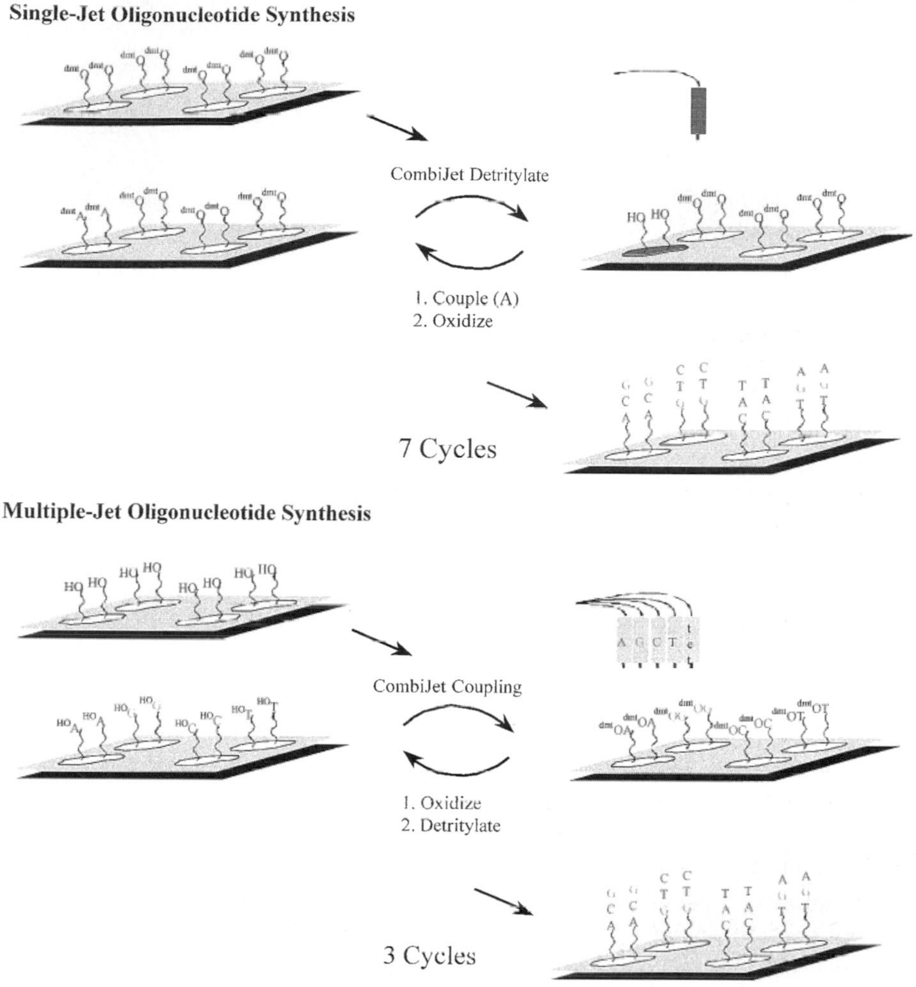

Single-Jet Oligonucleotide Synthesis

CombiJet Detritylate

1. Couple (A)
2. Oxidize

7 Cycles

Multiple-Jet Oligonucleotide Synthesis

CombiJet Coupling

1. Oxidize
2. Detritylate

3 Cycles

Figure 3. Synthesis of oligonucleotide arrays using CombiJet instruments. The upper diagram illustrates the synthesis of 3-mers using a single jet system. Seven synthesis cycles are required to complete the array. In the lower diagram the same 3-mer is synthesized utilizing a multiple jet system. In this case, three synthesis cycles are required to complete the array.

trol a set of valves that primes the jet. A strobe light and video monitoring system are used to ensure that the jet is operating correctly. For deprotection of specific regions on the surface of the slide, a program controls the x, y motion of the slide and the timing of firing of the jet. After deprotection is complete, the slide is rotated into a vertical orientation and moved to a wash station where the deprotection reagent is rinsed off the surface. At this point the slide is pushed onto a liquid flow chamber sealed by an o-ring. Reactions

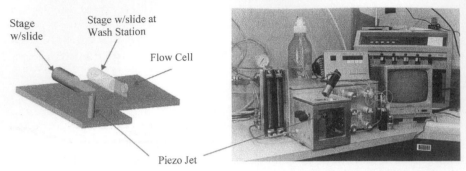

Figure 4. CombiJet schematic and photograph. For simplicity, the schematic has been drawn without most of the hardware. The stage is attached to x, y, and θ motion axes and positions the synthesis substrate over the jet, at the wash station, or at the flow cell.

for phosphoramidite base coupling and oxidation are then performed in a manner similar to that of an automated oligonucleotide synthesizer. During synthesis, the microscope slide remains in a chamber that can be sealed from the atmosphere and filled with anhydrous gas.

The operation of the instrument is fully controlled by a Windows program. Given a set of oligonucleotide sequences, automated routines lay out the pattern of jet firing for each cycle of synthesis. The various elemental steps of the synthesis cycle can either be controlled directly by an operator or linked together in text-based macros. This allows the complete synthesis of the molecular arrays with no further operator intervention.

3.3 Testing synthesis yield

One daunting aspect of the *in situ* DNA microarray synthesis is the fact that no purification of the synthesized material is possible. All products and by-products of synthesis remain attached to the surface. The quality of the material in each locus is thus determined by the stepwise coupling efficiency. In order to evaluate the coupling yield, a set of 64 spots of identical sequence was synthesized with a cleavable attachment to the surface. At the end of 15 cycles, the slide was subjected to a gas phase base reaction to disrupt the surface attachment. The oligos were collected by washing the surface. After complete removal of the remaining protecting groups, the oligo product was end-labelled with ^{32}P phosphate and subjected to polyacrylamide gel electrophoresis. By quantitatively analysing the banding pattern of the oligo products, it was possible to derive the average stepwise yield of the reactions. A stepwise yield of 91% was obtained.

The above experiment is expected to underestimate the coupling efficiency in the centre of a synthesis locus. Since the droplets do not occupy the same exact positions from cycle to cycle in the synthesis, the area in the fringe region of the locus will have an indeterminate history of reagents. For a locus of 200 μm, an offset of 10 μm from one cycle to the next will result in a non-overlapping region with 7.4% of the area of the spot. Shortened products will definitely accumulate in this region. Thus, it is anticipated that the central region of the locus has a much higher stepwise synthesis yield.

3.4 Linkers used for *in situ* synthesis

In order to maximize hybridization to the solid phase bound DNA, the amount of DNA attached to the surface as well as its availability for hybridization must be optimized. Linkers must be chosen such that the oligonucleotide synthesis can proceed efficiently while simultaneously providing the necessary spacing for effective hybridization in an aqueous hybridization mixture (11).

In order to evaluate the effect of linker length on hybridization, oligonucleotides were synthesized on polyethylene glycol polymers of various lengths. Labelled oligonucleotides were prepared with various lengths. An exact match 15-mer and a 50 base pair oligo containing the exact match at the 3′ end were constructed. In this configuration, the overhanging 25 base pairs are directed at the surface in order to create steric crowding. Results of hybridization experiments with these oligos and the surface bound oligos on the various PEG linker lengths were compared. For each linker length, the ratio of hybridization intensity of the 50-mer to the 15-mer was calculated. The ratio significantly improved as longer lengths of linker were used. It is anticipated that these longer linkers will assist in hybridization when complex mixtures of labelled samples are used.

3.5 Solvents for jetting

One of the more difficult aspects of using ink-jet technology for organic synthesis is finding solvents that are compatible both with the ink-jet hardware and the particular chemical reactions desired. In the case of oligonucleotide synthesis, acetonitrile is commonly used as a solvent for the phosphoramidites (12, 13). For the deprotection reagent, di- or trichloroacetic acid is typical. These solvents are quite volatile and do not represent the optimal choice for the ink-jet approach.

For the single jet device, we needed to adapt the deprotection step. The trichloroacetic acid reagent was too volatile for localized deprotection. An alternative Lewis acid-based method had been used previously to remove dimethoxytrityl protecting groups for oligonucleotide synthesis. One of the reported reagents was zinc bromide in a solvent mixture of dichloromethane and isopropanol (14). This reagent was expected to be much better for localized deprotection due to the non-volatility of the acid reagent. The less volatile dibromomethane was used to replace the dichloromethane. Tests in synthesizing oligonucleotides on beads in a synthesizer showed little difference between this zinc bromide-based reagent and the standard trichloroacetic acid mixture. The zinc bromide, dibromomethane/isopropanol reagent was thus very effective in removing the dimethoxytrityl protecting group and could be delivered reliably with the jet device. Ultimately a less volatile alcohol was substituted for isopropanol to prevent clogging of the jet with precipitated zinc bromide.

Adapting a solvent or chemical system to ensure adequate performance with the ink-jet approach can likely be done for a wide variety of chemical synthesis methods. In many cases, alternative synthetic approaches with solvent systems that are much more compatible with ink-jet delivery have already been reported in the literature. Adding co-solvents to the reagent that overcome the limitations of a particular solvent system is also possible. In either case, care must be taken to ensure that the change in a chemical reagent or solvent does not adversely affect the yield of the desired reaction.

3.6 CombiJet advantages

There are two main advantages of the CombiJet approach. The first is flexibility. Any combination of oligonucleotides, including varied lengths and mixtures at particular loci, can be generated using this device. Since the instrument is using 'off-the-shelf' chemistry for the most part, new advances in the field of oligonucleotide synthesis can be applied directly. This is particularly useful where backbone modifications or nucleotide base substitutions can be used to enhance the performance characteristics of the microarray. A further advantage is the fact that a variety of substrates can be used as the printing targets. This allows for porous membranes or other flow-through systems to be generated with DNA microarrays attached. One application that takes advantage of the system's flexibility is the parallel synthesis of oligonucleotides in preparative quantities. In cases where a defined mixture of oligonucleotide targets is desired, the CombiJet is a very effective instrument for their synthesis.

The second advantage of the CombiJet system is its low cost for the production of DNA microarrays. This is especially true for the mode of printing where phosphoramidites are delivered by the jets. In this case, the greatest cost for synthesis comes from the acetonitrile and other solvents used to rinse the array between the chemical steps. Phosphoramidites, which typically represent the majority of cost and oligonucleotide synthesis (excluding purification), are used so effectively that, at current prices, less than ten cents worth of phosphoramidites would be required for the generation of an array of 10 000 15-mers.

3.7 Critical technology issues

In order to move from the research phase into DNA microarray synthesis of commercial scale, certain key technology improvements will be required. The cycle time of the instrument is approximately ten minutes, relatively independent of the number of elements within the array. This means an array of 18-

mers takes three hours to print. Obviously, the next generation instrument will need to print on more than one array at a time. The batch production mode will allow functional-based sampling of arrays to be included as the quality assurance measure.

Other issues to be addressed are the robustness of jetting and the reduction of jet-to-jet variability. Improvements in jet manufacturing have allowed great strides in this area. However, even small differences in orifice size or the geometry of the glass leading into the orifice can have a profound effect on the volume of drop generated, the degree of satellite formation, and the droplet trajectory as it leaves the orifice. Presently a skilled operator is required to tailor the driving pulse of the jets to ensure that droplet generation meets expectations.

Another area where significant improvement can be made is in changing from the uniform glass substrate to a surface with a pattern defining the zones where synthesis will occur or a surface with porosity. The patterned regions would be effective at reducing or eliminating the 'fringe' region of the synthesis loci where uncontrolled chemical delivery occurs. This would improve and normalize the synthesis yield over the entire locus. The porous substrate would be beneficial in increasing the surface area and hence the number of oligonucleotides synthesized.

4. Molecular array fabrication by deposition

From the standpoint of droplet generation, deposition of pre-synthesized biological material is much like the native printing mode of the ink-jet technology. In the case of deposition of DNA and other biomolecules, the material can be supplied in an aqueous buffer, much like some of the inks used in printing. However, as mentioned above, the main issue is not only drop generation, but in accessing a very large number of different samples. Further, the DNA samples are moderately expensive to generate and must be kept at high concentration for reaction with the solid phase. Thus small quantities of the liquid are available to carry out the filling and priming of the jets. The Gene-Jet series of instruments was designed to take advantage of the piezoelectric capillary jet's ability to generate small precisely placed droplets at high speed. Due to the small size of the capillary, the jet is loaded by aspirating DNA containing aqueous samples from microtitre plates. In order to efficiently use the sample material, a large platter was provided to carry multiple glass microscope slides. A more detailed description of the device follows.

4.1 GeneJet instrument description

A schematic and a photograph of the GeneJet III device are presented in *Figure 5*. The device is designed to use up to eight jets to aspirate samples from 384- or 1536-well microtitre plates and apply them to microarrays. Five

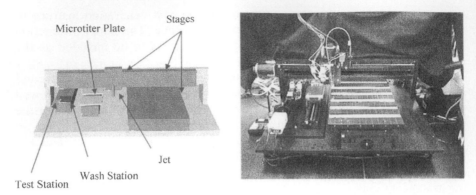

Figure 5. GeneJet schematic and photograph.

independent axes exist on the instrument. A high speed x axis carries a z axis onto which the print head is mounted. Three axes of motion rest under the x, z arrangement. A print platter that holds up to 96 glass microscope slides using a vacuum chuck to maintain their positions is mounted on the y axis. The platter is extremely flat with a total deviation in height, as seen by the jet, of about 20 µm. This allows the jet-to-surface distance to be minimized to ensure accurate drop placement. The u axis carries cleaning, washing, and test firing stations. A pair of microtitre plates holding reagents are secured to the v axis with individual vacuum chucks.

Each of the jets is independently connected to a set of solenoid valves that control aspiration of DNA containing samples as well as aspiration of liquids used for the cleaning cycle. In cases where fewer than 2000 drops are required, the jet can be pre-filled with water and then a 1–2 µl plug of the DNA containing sample can be loaded. This minimizes the amount of material required for printing. On the order of 2000 drops can be printed before dilution of the sample is seen.

The test firing area is monitored by a video camera. An operator can visualize the droplets to ensure that the jet has been successfully loaded with sample material and is delivering droplets free from satellites. If required, adjustment of the voltage waveform can be made. The test firing area can also be monitored by automated software to determine if drops are being delivered. The software captures an image frame from the video both before and after a single pulse of the jet. The two frames are compared to determine if a droplet has been delivered.

Two modes of printing are available. The first mode, 'start-stop', is characterized by the jet positioning in x, y, and z relative to a point on the platter, stopping all motion and subsequently firing. In this mode, one or more droplets can be placed at a specific location. The second mode of printing, 'print-on-the-fly', offers much higher throughput. In this case, the jet moves to the start of a print line in the x, y, and z coordinates and then continues to move in x alone to reach the end of the print line. The placement of drops is performed by timing the firing of the jet to its location in the print line. Software routines pre-calculate the print line and fill a buffer with fire commands that are calculated based upon the jet's position. Because the rate of firing of jets is high compared to the average time for travel between points to be printed, the time required to print drops on a line of arrays is the same no matter how may drops occur on that line. Furthermore, no additional time is required for multiple jets to print on the same line.

4.2 Software

The software used to run the instrument is extremely flexible and takes full advantage of the capabilities of the hardware. The user interacts with the device through a Windows control program. As with CombiJet, the user can directly manipulate all elemental movements or procedural routines of the instrument and can further combine these elemental operations together in powerful macros to accomplish completely automated printing of micro-arrays. At the start of the batch run, the operator enters or loads a list which indexes a set of genes and provides their location in the microtitre plate wells. An array template file is then associated with one or more positions on a platter where that array is to be printed. Multiple array template files can be used on the same print platter as long as all of the genes are available in the microtitre plates. The platter layout is also flexible in that any number of arrays can be printed on the platter, provided they do not physically overlap each other. Thus, in addition to printing single arrays on microscope slides, wafers of glass with multiple arrays can be generated.

4.3 DNA microarrays manufactured by GeneJet

An example of an array printed with the GeneJet instrument is shown in *Figure 6*. Based on the concentration of material and the expected amount of cross-linking to the surface, 5–50 attomoles of material are available in each spot. No shearing of DNA strands has been observed with material up to 2000 base pairs in length. To date, the instrument has not been used for longer pieces of DNA, however, it is anticipated that viscosity will place a practical limit on the length of DNA that can be jetted effectively with the piezo capillary jets. This is due to the fact that in the preferred mode, the DNA needs to be concentrated enough that a single drop deposits the desired amount of material in an array locus. At the desired concentrations (1 μg/μl), DNA of 5 kb and larger will likely be too viscous for a small (30 μm) orifice jet. Viscosity reduction by adding co-solvents may help to some extent.

4.4 Reproducibility in spotting

To determine the intrinsic variability in spotting, nine dsDNA samples were loaded and spotted repeatedly. The array was processed and then treated with

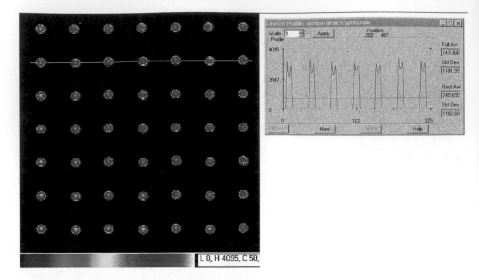

Figure 6. GeneJet array. Fluorescently labelled DNA was spotted using GeneJet III. The spots are ~150 μm in diameter with a centre-to-centre spacing of 508 μm. A profile of the fluorescence intensity across a scan line is shown.

a dsDNA fluorescent stain. The standard deviation of the integrated spot intensities was 13% of its average. Similar results have been obtained in experiments where pre-labelled DNA was spotted. It must be noted that although these experiments attempt to isolate the printing process, the variability estimates obtained are a convolution of the variability in spotting, surface non-uniformity, the variability in fluorescence intensity, and the variability in detection. Fluorescence intensity is greatly effected by the local environment of the fluorophore and quenching. Variation in the surface chemical environment or local density of material could thus have a significant and non-linear effect.

4.5 Critical technology issues

An enhancement in throughput can be achieved by utilizing multiple jets while retaining the print-on-the-fly mode of operation. As discussed in the next section, a multiple jet system is needed to keep pace with other modes of depositing DNA in microarrays. Thus, like CombiJet, the main issues in using GeneJet as a manufacturing tool are jet robustness and jet-to-jet reproducibility. This becomes especially important for a multiple jet instrument. Although the instrument can support distinct waveforms for each jet, it would be preferable to improve jet manufacture to the point where a common waveform could be supplied to all jets to generate droplets of precisely the same size, free of satellites, and propagating at the same velocity.

114

4.6 Advantages of the GeneJet approach

4.6.1 Deposition devices: contact versus non-contact

A comparison of contact and non-contact printing will reveal one of the key advantages of the ink-jet approach: speed in printing. The calculations which follow are directed at the difference that exists between the jet approach and what will be broadly classified as 'pin tools'. For the purpose of this calculation, 'pin tools' will refer to any printing method where a liquid reagent delivery tip needs to be brought into close proximity with a surface to deliver an aliquot of liquid. Typically this will involve a vertical motion that touches the tip to the surface to leave behind a droplet of the liquid material. During this vertical motion, horizontal motion is stopped. This is the root of the difference between non-contact and contact modes of printing. Since motion must stop for each contact, the time to print a batch of arrays grows linearly with the number of arrays in the batch. In contrast, for non-contact printing methods operating in the 'print-on-the-fly' mode, horizontal motion does not need to stop in order to deliver aliquots of liquid. The time to print a batch of arrays increases much more slowly with batch size. Further, as will be shown, this result is independent of the number of different genes printed.

4.6.2 Batch print time

The total time to print a batch of arrays includes the set up time, the time spent cleaning and loading the liquid deposition devices, and the print time itself:

$$\text{total time} = \text{print time} + \text{fill time} + \text{set up time}.$$

Print time includes all time associated with movement and deposition of spots. Fill time includes all wash steps for the deposition device, time for loading the device, and time for testing the load and getting into position for printing. Set up time includes the time to load the array substrates and microtitre plates, etc. containing array element material as well as time to offload the instrument when the batch run in complete. For either the pin or the jet instruments, the sum of print time and fill time can be expressed in terms of the number of instrument cycles and the time per cycle for each component:

print time + fill time = (number of cycles) $\times$ (print time/cycle + fill time/cycle).

Thus we have:

$$T = C\,(PT_{cyc} + T_f) + T_s \qquad\qquad [1]$$

where T = total time, C = cycles, PT_{cyc} = print time per cycle, T_f = fill time per cycle, T_s = set up time.
  For the pin tool:

$$PT_{cyc} = NT_c$$

where N = number of arrays printed, T_c = contact time per array including motion.

$$C = G/P$$

where G = number of genes, P = number of pins.

Combining terms, the total print time for a batch mode pin device is thus:

$$Tp = G/P \, (NTc + Tf,p) + Ts,p \tag{2}$$

For the jet instrument:

$$Ptcyc = RTl$$
$$C = G/J$$

where R = number of rows of arrays on a platter, Tl = print time per line, J = number of jets.

If the set of arrays to be printed is arranged in a square, then the number of rows will be given by:

$$R = \sqrt{N}$$

Combining the above terms, the total time for batch printing with the jet approach is:

$$Tj = G/J \, (vR \, Tl + Tf,j) + Ts,j \tag{3}$$

Inspection of *Equations 2* and *3* reveals the key aspects of the two printing approaches. In both cases, reduction of the set up time will lead to corresponding reduction in the total time to process a batch of arrays. This is especially important for a small number of cycles. In terms of printing a large number of genes, a huge reduction in time can be achieved by multiplying the number of printing tools to reduce the number of cycles of printing.

The main difference between the two approaches is that the time for printing with the jet approach depends on the number of rows of arrays whereas that of the pin approach depends simply on the number of arrays. For large numbers of arrays, the batch print time for the jet instrument becomes dependent on the square root of the number of arrays as opposed to growing linearly with the number of arrays as is the case for the pin tool.

It is possible to place realistic values on some of the parameters in *Equations 2* and *3* in order to estimate what is most important in practice. The time required to set up a typical instrument will be roughly 30 minutes. During the cycle, the time required to fill either the pen or ink-jet device will be about 40 seconds. This time includes a cleaning procedure that is required to prepare the device for the next material to be spotted. For the jet device, an additional 20 seconds is required to ensure that it is properly primed for printing. The

Table 2. Time estimates

Step	Time
Ts,p; Ts,j	30 min
Tf,p	40 sec
Tf,j	60 sec
Tc	0.75 sec
Tl	1 sec

Table 3. Batch times (hours)

Arrays	Genes	Jets				Pins			
		1	4	16	96	4	16	96	384
100	100	2.4	1.0	0.6	0.5	1.3	0.7	0.5	0.5
	1000	20	5.4	1.7	0.7	8.5	2.5	0.8	0.6
	10 000	190	49	13	2.5	80	21	3.8	1.3
	100 000	1900	490	120	21	800	200	34	8.8
1000	100	3.0	1.1	0.7	0.5	6.0	1.9	0.7	0.6
	1000	26	6.9	2.1	0.8	55	14	2.8	1.1
	10 000	260	64	16	3.2	550	140	23	6.2
	100 000	2500	640	160	27	5500	1400	230	58
10 000	100	4.9	1.6	0.8	0.5	53	14	2.7	1.0
	1000	45	12	3.3	1.0	520	130	22	6.0
	10 000	440	110	28	5.1	5200	1300	220	55
	100 000	4400	1100	280	47	52 000	13 000	2200	550

contact time for the pen device will vary among instruments, but a rate of one to two contacts per second is realistic. Finally, the time per line of print on the jet instrument can be estimated as one per second. *Table 2* summarizes these time estimates.

Using the values in *Table 2* and in *Equations 2* and *3*, it is possible to compare the total print time for various configurations of the pen and jet instruments. *Table 3* and *Figures 7* and *8* show the results of the calculations for various instrument configurations, array complexities, and batch sizes. If the number of jets and pens is equal, the jet instrument will always have the time advantage. However, since it is generally easier to multiplex pins than jets, the pin instrument will have an advantage for small batch sizes. Such advantage will be lost as batch size increases. For any particular configuration in terms of the number of jets or pins, the cross-over point is independent of the number of genes printed. This can be seen by finding the point as a function of the number of arrays where the total print times are equal.

Setting *Equation 2* equal to *Equation 3*:

$$G/P \, (NTc + Tf,p) + Ts,p = G/J \, (RTl + Tf,j) + Ts,j$$

we see that for large N the number of genes factors out of the solution for N. This point is further illustrated in *Figures 7* and *8*.

4.6.3 Flexibility

An advantage of the non-contact mode of printing is its flexibility. In principle, the pattern of drop delivery to surfaces can be completely configured in the software of the instrument. There is no major constraint placed on the size of the array or placement of drops due to constraints such as loading from a microtitre plate. In other words, even though jets must go into the microtitre

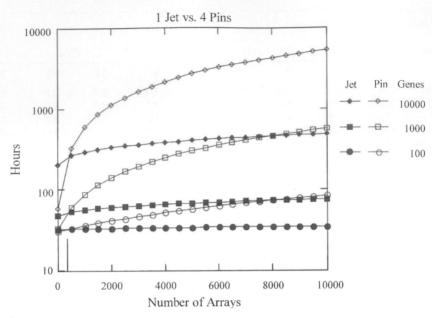

Figure 7. Batch print time comparison for one jet and four pin instruments. Various array complexities in terms of the number of different array elements are shown. As the number of arrays increases, the time required to print with the pin instrument increases faster than that of the jet instrument. Independent of the number of genes printed, both systems take the same amount of time to print 370 arrays.

plate at, for example, the standard 9 mm spacing, since delivery of droplets is done by timing the firing of jets, placement of drops from adjacent jets is not constrained to a 9 mm spacing. Thus, large objects such as microtitre plates can be mapped onto much smaller formats. In addition, this printing programmability allows for placement of drops on pre-configured substrates. This is especially important when a detection system or other component of that assay requires fixed locations of array elements.

5. Conclusion

The application of the ink-jet technology to the manufacture of DNA microarrays has been demonstrated. The *in situ* approach provides great flexibility and low cost in the production of massively parallel oligonucleotide arrays. Current stepwise coupling yields are adequate for the production of arrays that can be used in a variety of diagnostic or research applications. In addition to standard microarrays, this approach offers a unique ability to synthesize preparative quantities of oligonucleotide products that can be detached from the solid phase substrate and used in biological assays.

The use of ink-jet technology in an instrument designed to deposit pre-

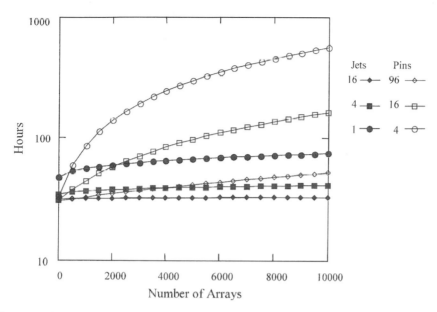

Figure 8. Comparison of print times for 1000 spot arrays with various instrument configurations. In all cases, the jet instrument is favoured for large number of arrays.

synthesized material has been demonstrated in a manufacturing prototype instrument. Several thousand arrays have been produced. The technology is most effective when large numbers of arrays are fabricated simultaneously. The combination of a multiple jet print head and the 'print-on-the-fly' mode of operation will be a winning solution in the manufacturing environment.

Acknowledgements

This work was partially supported by a grant from the US Department of Commerce/National Institute of Standards and Technology under the Advanced Technology Program Tools for DNA Diagnostics (94-05). John Blanchard wrote the majority of control software used for the GeneJet and CombiJet instruments. The authors wish to thank Ai Ching Lim, Sang Park, Terence Flynn, Tim Johann, Jennifer Cormack, Jon McDunn, Winters Reef Hardy, and John Baldeschwieler for their contributions to the projects described herein. The authors also thank Christine Coleman for a critical reading of this manuscript.

References

1. Blanchard, A. P., Kaiser, R. J., and Hood, L. E. (1996). *Biosens. Bio.*, **11**, 687.
2. Schena, M., Heller, R. A., Theriault, T. P., Konrad, K., Lachenmeier, E., and Davis, R. W. (1998). *Trends Biotechnol.*, **16**, 301.

3. Bugdayci, N., Bogy, D. B., and Talke, F. E. (1983). *IBM J. Res. Dev.*, **27**, 171.
4. Adams, R. L. and Roy, J. (1986). *J. Appl. Mech.*, **53**, 193.
5. Shield, T. W., Bogy, D. B., and Talke, F. E. (1987). *IBM J. Res. Dev.*, **31**, 96.
6. Asai, A. (1992). *J. Fluids Eng.*, **114**, 638.
7. Peeters, E. and Verdonckt-Vandebrock, S. (1997). *IEEE-Circ. Dev.*, **13**, 19.
8. Tam, A. C. and Gill, W. D. (1982). *Appl. Opt.*, **21**, 1891.
9. Elrod, S. A., Hadimioglu, B., Khuri-Yakub, B. T., Rawson, E. G., Richley, E., Quate, C. F., *et al.* (1989). *J. Appl. Phys.*, **65**, 3441.
10. Hadimiogly, B., Elrod, S. A., Steinmetz, D. L., Lim, M., Zesch, J. C., Khuri-Yakub, B. T., *et al.* (1992). *Ultrasonics Symp.*, 929.
11. Maskos, U. and Southern, E. M. (1992). *Nucleic Acids Res.*, **20**, 1679.
12. Gait, M. J. (1984). *Oligonucleotide synthesis: a practical approach.* IRL Press, Oxford.
13. Beaucage, S. L. and Iyer, R. P. (1992). *Tetrahedron*, **48**, 2223.
14. Kierzek, R. H., Ito, R. B., and Itakura, K. (1981). *Tetrahedron Lett.*, **22**, 3761.

7

Gene expression analysis via cDNA microarrays of laser capture microdissected cells from fixed tissue

RANELLE C. SALUNGA, HONGQING GUO, LIN LUO, ANTON BITTNER, K. C. JOY, JIM R. CHAMBERS, JACKSON S. WAN, MICHAEL R. JACKSON, and MARK G. ERLANDER

1. Introduction

The enormous number of DNA and mRNA sequences available to researchers, coupled with cDNA microarray technology, now allows for gene expression to be studied on a massive scale. Using microarrays, thousands of genes from organisms such as *S. cerevisiae* (1, 2) and *A. thaliana* (3), as well as those from mammalian species (4), have been analysed. However, most methods that have been described to date have relied on acquiring microgram quantities of messenger RNA or poly(A) RNA from pure populations of cells, in order to synthesize cDNA probes (1–6).

This technical requirement of isolating large amounts of mRNA severely limits the study of gene expression from individual cell types within a given organ, tissue, or system. A recent technology, laser capture microdissection (LCM), now gives the researcher the ability to procure specific cell types from a given tissue section (7). The great advantage that LCM provides is that it allows single-cell resolution of the tissue being analysed, and thus enables the researcher the ability to capture discrete cells (see *Figure 1*). Because relatively small numbers of cells are usually captured, it is necessary to perform an RNA amplification step prior to probe synthesis. We present here protocols that integrate the use of LCM, RNA amplification, and cDNA microarrays for studying gene expression at the cellular level.

2. Laser capture microdissection

The LCM technique was originally invented at the NIH (8) and as part of a Collaborative Research and Development Agreement with Arcturus Engineering,

Ranelle C. Salunga et al.

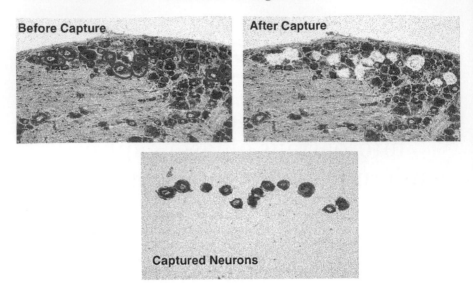

Figure 1. Laser capture of large DRG neurones. Upper left panel shows circled large DRG neurones that are targeted for laser capture. Upper right panel shows cells successfully transferred to film (lower panel) (18).

Inc., a commercially available instrument was developed. To capture cells from fixed tissue, a tissue section is mounted on a slide and viewed under an inverted microscope. A transparent cap, which fits into a 0.5 ml microcentrifuge tube, has attached to it a transfer film that is placed directly above the tissue to be examined. The cells of interest are then selected by activating a laser beam. The cells that are in the path of the laser beam become focally adhesive. The cells fuse to the transfer film by thermal adhesion and are lifted off for processing. RNA and DNA can then be extracted from the sample for further analysis. A more detailed description on LCM is available electronically (9).

2.1 Preparation of tissues for LCM
When handling tissue samples for RNA analysis and LCM, it is very important to observe laboratory practices that minimize and/or eliminate the possibility of RNase contamination. Gloves are to be worn at all times and solutions are prepared using H_2O treated with diethyl pyrocarbonate (DEPC). Further guidelines for working with RNA are adequately described elsewhere (10). The preservation of the RNA in these tissue samples is critical; improper handling usually leads to unsuccessful RNA amplification due to the compromised integrity of the total RNA extracted from the tissue.

122

Protocol 1. Tissue preparation and histological staining

It is critical to observe RNase-free conditions when preparing tissues.

Equipment and reagents

- Baked forceps and sterile scalpels
- Cryomould and OCT tissue embedding medium (Miles, Inc.)
- Plain glass slides, slide boxes, slide holders, staining dishes (VWR)
- Cryostat (Leica brand; McBain Instruments)
- Haematoxylin (Biogenex), eosin, and Bluing Reagent (Shandon)
- Xylene, ethanol, RNase-free water (United States Biochemical)

Method

1. Dissect fresh tissue using sterile, baked forceps and sterile scalpels. Place the tissue in a cryomould, cover it with OCT frozen tissue embedding medium, and then immerse it immediately in dry ice-cold 2-methylbutane at about −50°C. Store the tissues at −70°C until processed for cutting.

2. Cut tissue sections at 7–10 μm on a cryostat and mount each section on a plain, uncoated glass slide. *Immediately* lay the slide on the cold stage in the cryostat or on a block of dry ice to keep the tissue section frozen.

3. Transfer the slides into a slide box inside the cryostat and do not let the tissue thaw. Store the slide box at −70°C. Alternatively, if the slides are to be processed immediately, proceed to step 4.

4. Load the slides into a slide holder and immerse them *immediately* into 100% ethanol for 1 min.

5. To rehydrate the tissues, dip the slides in 95% ethanol, 70% ethanol, 50% ethanol, and in RNase-free H_2O, 12 times for each solution.

6. Stain the tissues in haematoxylin[a] for 15 sec. Dip the slides 12 times in RNase-free H_2O.

7. Dip the slides in Bluing Reagent for 30 sec and rinse them with RNase-free H_2O.

8. Stain the slides once in eosin Y for 10 sec and rinse them with RNase-free H_2O.

9. Dehydrate the slides by dipping them in 50% ethanol, 70% ethanol, 95% ethanol, and 100% ethanol, 12 times each.

10. Dip the slides slowly in xylene, about 12 times within a 1 min interval.

11. Shake off excess xylene and wipe the slides carefully with a particle-free tissue and air dry them for 10 min.

12. The slides are now ready for laser capture microdissection.

[a] For most tissues, use haematoxylin/eosin. For neuronal tissues, substitute Nissl stain for haematoxylin in step 6 and omit steps 7 and 8. Also, note that some tissues may require longer or shorter than 15 sec (this needs to be determined empirically).

2.2 Laser capture of fresh frozen specimens

The instrument we used for laser capture microdissection is the PixCell™ LCM System from Arcturus Engineering, Inc. A more thorough description of this instrument is available on the company website (9) and on the NIH website (11), where protocols for sample capture are discussed in detail.

2.3 RNA amplification

The necessity of an RNA amplification scheme to obtain sufficient material from limited LCM specimens is obvious. While it may be feasible to create representative cDNA libraries by PCR (12, 13), there is always a concern that PCR will lead to the preferential amplification of certain cDNAs and to variability from one reaction to another. For example, the exponential nature of PCR makes it rather arduous to determine the point at which linear amplification is achieved, particularly if many samples from multiple sources are to be analysed. RNA amplification via T7 RNA polymerase circumvents these problems because the amplification is linear rather than exponential as in the case of PCR.

RNA amplification involving T7 polymerase was first described as a tool for analysing gene expression in cerebellar tissues (14) and subsequently, in single, live rat hippocampus neurones (15). We have shown that cDNA probes

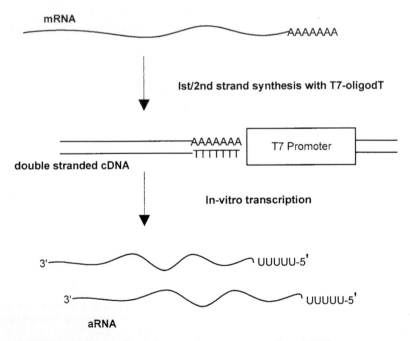

Figure 2. RNA amplification from the poly(A) component of total RNA.

synthesized from amplified RNA display similar hybridization patterns (on reverse Northern blots) as do cDNA probes synthesized from non-amplified, poly(A) RNA (16). The scheme for amplifying RNA with T7 polymerase is shown in *Figure 2*. The method relies on attaching a T7 promoter sequence to the oligo(dT) primer used for synthesis of the first cDNA strand. After second strand cDNA synthesis, one can generate amplified RNA (aRNA) using T7 RNA polymerase and the double-stranded cDNA molecules as targets for the linear amplification.

2.4 RNA extraction

While this chapter focuses specifically on LCM samples, RNA amplification can be used on any tissue or cell sample in which the RNA is present in small quantities. Total RNA extracted with commercially available RNA preparation reagents such as Trizol (Gibco), RNAzol B (Tel Test, Inc.), or RNeasy (Qiagen) are suitable for extractions with bulk tissue samples. However, the RNA needs to be free of contaminating genomic DNA as pointed out in Section 3.

Protocol 2. Extraction of total RNA from LCM samples

Reagents
- Micro RNA isolation kit (Stratagene)
- Glycogen (Boehringer Mannheim)
- RNasin (Promega)
- DNase I (Genhunter)
- RNase-free H_2O (United States Biochemical)

Method[a]

1. Determine the total amount of denaturing solution (provided in the kit) needed and prepare it by adding 7.2 μl 2-mercaptoethanol/ml. Each LCM sample requires 200 μl denaturing solution.

2. Add 200 μl denaturing buffer solution into each tube and mix by inverting the tubes and by gentle vortexing. Incubate the tubes at room temperature for 5 min to allow the cells to dissolve in the solution.

3. Centrifuge each tube for a few seconds and transfer the contents to a 1.5 ml Eppendorf tube. Add 20 μl 2 M sodium acetate, 220 μl phenol, and 60 μl chloroform:isoamyl alcohol. Vortex the tubes vigorously for 30 sec and incubate the samples on ice for 5 min.

4. Spin the samples at 4°C at 14000 r.p.m. for 5 min in a microcentrifuge. Collect and transfer the aqueous layer to a new tube.

5. Add 1 μl 10 mg/ml glycogen and 200 μl isopropanol. Mix the contents of the tubes by inversion and incubate them at –70°C for 15 min.

6. Centrifuge the tubes at 4°C at 14000 r.p.m. for 30 min in a microcentrifuge. Remove the supernatant taking care not to disrupt the pellet.

Protocol 2. *Continued*

7. Wash the RNA pellet with cold 75% ethanol.[b] Centrifuge the tubes briefly for 5 min at 14 000 r.p.m in a microcentrifuge.

8. Remove the supernatant and air dry the RNA pellet.

9. Resuspend the pellet in 16 μl RNase-free H_2O, 2 μl 10 × DNase I reaction buffer,[c] 1 μl RNasin, and 1 μl DNase I. Incubate the tubes at 37°C for 30 min.

10. Add 2 μl 2 M sodium acetate, 22 μl phenol, and 6 μl chloroform. Vortex the tubes vigorously and incubate the samples on ice for 5 min. Repeat steps 4–7 of this protocol.

11. Resuspend the pellet in 11 μl. Remove 1 μl and use this as a negative control in the reverse transcription (RT) reaction (see *Protocol 3*). This will be your no RT control. Use the remaining 10 μl the reverse transcription reaction in *Protocol 3*.

12. Freeze RNA at −70°C.

---

[a] Manufacturer's protocol with a few modifications.
[b] 75% ethanol should be made with RNase-free H_2O.
[c] 10 × DNase I reaction buffer: 100 mM Tris pH 8.4, 15 mM $MgCl_2$, 500 mM KCl, and 0.01% gelatin.

3. Generation of aRNA—first round

One can make amplified RNA from any preparation of total RNA. It is important that the RNA used for this procedure is free from contaminating DNA. Therefore, it is necessary to pre-treat the RNA preparation with DNase I prior to starting RT–PCR (*Protocol 2*, step 9). The steps used for the first round of RNA amplification are described in *Protocol 3*.

Protocol 3. Amplifying RNA from total RNA—first and second strand syntheses

Equipment and reagents

- Superscript Choice System for cDNA synthesis (Gibco)
- HPLC purified T7 oligo(dT) primer (Operon): 5′-TCTAGTCGACGGCCAGTGAATTGTAAT-ACGACTCACTATAGGGCG(T)$_{21}$-3′
- Microcon-100 columns (Millipore)
- RNasin (Promega)
- RNase-free H_2O (United States Biochemical)

Method

1. Obtain the 10 μl RNA sample from *Protocol 2*, step 12. Add 1 μl 0.5 mg/ml T7 oligo(dT) primer.

2. Heat the samples at 70°C for 10 min. Chill them on ice immediately. Spin down each sample by centrifugation in a microcentrifuge.

3. Equilibrate each tube at 42°C for 5 min.

4. Add 4 μl 5 × first strand buffer,[a] 2 μl 0.1 M DTT, 1 μl 10 mM dNTPs, 1 μl RNasin, and 1 μl Superscript RI II.

5. Incubate the tubes at 42°C for 60 min.

6. Remove 1 μl and perform PCR as described in Section 3.1.

7. To the remainder of the first strand reaction, add 30 μl second strand synthesis buffer,[b] 3 μl 10 mM dNTPs, 4 μl DNA polymerase I, 1 μl *E. coli* RNase H, 1 μl *E. coli* DNA ligase, and 92 μl RNase-free H_2O.

8. Mix the contents gently by pipetting and incubate at 16°C for 2 h.

9. Add 2 μl T4 DNA polymerase. Incubate at 16°C for 10 min.

10. Extract samples once with phenol:chloroform (1:1, v/v) and collect aqueous layer.

11. To remove unincorporated nucleotides and salts, prepare Microcon-100 columns by pre-rinsing with 500 μl RNase-free H_2O. Spin at room temperature for about 12–15 min at 500 *g*.

12. Load each sample onto a Microcon-100 column and bring up the volume in the column to 500 μl. Spin the columns at 500 *g* for 12–15 min at room temperature.

13. Perform two more rinses with 500 μl RNase-free H_2O, each time spinning at 500 *g* for about 12–15 min.[c]

14. Invert each column into a 1.5 ml collection tube and collect the samples by brief centrifugation.

15. Reduce the sample volume to 8 μl by vacuum centrifugation.

16. Proceed with *Protocol 4* (*in vitro* transcription).

[a] 5 × first strand buffer: 250 mM Tris–HCl pH 8.3, 375 mM KCl, 15 mM $MgCl_2$.
[b] 5 × second strand buffer: 100 mM Tris–HCl pH 6.9, 450 mM KCl, 23 mM $MgCl_2$, 0.75 mM βNAD⁺, 50 mM $(NH_4)_2SO_4$.
[c] Monitor the Microcon-100 columns and avoid drying. Centrifugation for > 15 min or at speeds greater than > 500 *g* may lead to column drying and sample loss.

3.1 PCR set up

The reverse transcription reaction for the RT–PCR is outlined in *Protocol 3*, steps 1–6. For a particular sample, the optimal analysis requires performing RT–PCR on several mRNAs with moderate (~ 1/1000) and low (< 1/10 000) expression level. For example, in brain samples, we use β-actin and neurone-specific enolase. Typically, 35–40 cycles are sufficient to generate a robust signal as measured by electrophoresis using agarose gels and ethidium bromide staining. For the PCR, transfer 1 μl from the first strand reaction into a PCR tube as described in *Protocol 3*, step 6. Add 5 μl 10 × PCR buffer (100 mM

Tris–HCl pH 8.3, 15 mM MgCl$_2$, 500 mM KCl, and 0.01% gelatin) (Perkin Elmer), 2.5 U *Taq* DNA polymerase (Perkin Elmer), 0.4 μl 25 mM dNTPs (Pharmacia), 25 pmol each of two primers, and bring up the volume of the reaction to 50 μl with sterile water. Perform cycling parameters for your primer set using established procedures (17). Run the PCR products in an agarose gel to assess whether intact RNA was successfully obtained.

3.2 Generating aRNA by *in vitro* transcription

Protocol 4. *In vitro* transcription and purification

When setting up the transcription reaction, make sure that all the components (except the T7 RNA polymerase) have been equilibrated to room temperature to prevent the irreversible precipitation of the cDNA caused by the presence of spermidine in the transcription buffer.

Equipment and reagents
- Ampliscribe T7 transcription kit (Epicentre Technologies)
- Microcon-100 (Millipore)

Method
1. Obtain the cDNA from *Protocol 3*, step 15. Make sure the cDNA is in a total volume of 8 μl.
2. Add 2 μl 10 × AmpliscribeT7 buffer.
3. Add 1.5 μl ATP, 1.5 μl CTP, 1.5 μl GTP, and 1.5 μl UTP in this order.
4. Add 2 μl 0.1 M DTT and mix.
5. Add 2 μl T7 RNA polymerase.
6. Alternatively, a master mix may be prepared if one is processing multiple samples, but the order in which reaction components in the master mix are assembled should be exactly as outlined in steps 2–5 of this protocol.
7. Incubate samples at 42°C for 3 h.
8. Add 1 μl RNase-free DNase (from the kit).
9. Incubate the samples at 37°C for 15 min.
10. Purify the aRNA using a Microcon-100 column as described in *Protocol 3*, steps 11–14.
11. Freeze the aRNA at –70°C. Alternatively, if you are going to re-amplify the aRNA, reduce the volume of the aRNA to 10 μl by vacuum centrifugation and proceed to *Protocol 5*.

When starting with at least 1 μg total RNA as the starting material in *Protocol 3*, there should be enough aRNA generated from a single round of transcription for cDNA probe synthesis. In our experience, we obtain 10–20 μg aRNA from 1–2 μg total RNA as starting material. If this is the case, proceed to *Protocol 7*, which outlines cDNA probe synthesis from aRNA. However, most total RNA preparations obtained from LCM samples yield only a few nanograms of total RNA; therefore, two to three rounds of amplification are needed to obtain enough aRNA for probe synthesis.

3.3 Generation of aRNA—subsequent rounds

The aRNA obtained from the first round of amplification is the antisense sequence relative to cDNA from which it was transcribed (*Figure 2*). To re-generate the T7 promoter sequence for use in subsequent rounds, one needs to prime the first strand cDNA synthesis reaction with random hexamers and generate second strand products. *Protocol 5* outlines how to regenerate double-stranded cDNA templates each containing a T7 promoter sequence.

Protocol 5.   Re-amplifying RNA from aRNA: first and second strand syntheses

Reagents

- Random hexamers (Pharmacia)
- Supercript Choice System for cDNA synthesis (Gibco)
- RNasin (Promega)
- RNase-free H_2O (United States Biochemical)

Method

1. Add 1 μl 1 mg/ml random hexamers to the aRNA obtained from *Protocol 4*, step 11.
2. Heat the samples at 70°C for 10 min. Chill the tubes on ice. Spin them briefly in a microcentrifuge.
3. Equilibrate the samples for 10 min at room temperature.
4. Add 4 μl 5 × first strand buffer, 2 μl 0.1 M DTT, 1 μl 10 mM dNTPs, 1 μl RNasin, and 1 μl Superscript RT II.
5. Incubate the samples at room temperature for 5 min.
6. Incubate the samples at 37°C for 1 h.
7. Add 1 μl RNase H to each tube. Mix gently.
8. Incubate the samples at 37°C for 20 min.[a]
9. Heat the samples at 95°C for 2 min to denature the hybrids.
10. Chill the samples on ice. Spin the samples briefly, and on ice add 1 μl 0.5 mg/ml T7 oligo(dT) primer.
11. Heat the samples to 70°C for 5 min, spin them very briefly in a micro-centrifuge, and then incubate them directly at 42°C for 10 min to

---

Protocol 5. *Continued*

anneal the T7 oligo(dT) primer. Chill the samples on ice. Spin the samples briefly.

12. Add 30 μl second strand synthesis buffer, 3 μl 10 mM dNTPs, 4 μl DNA polymerase I, 1 μl RNase H, and 90 μl RNase-free H_2O.

13. Incubate the samples at 16°C for 2 h.

14. Add 2 μl T4 DNA polymerase. Mix gently. Incubate the samples at 16°C for 10 min.

15. Add 150 μl phenol:chloroform. Vortex the samples for about 10 sec.

16. Spin the samples at 12 000 *g* in a microcentrifuge. Take the aqueous layer and transfer it to a new tube.

17. Purify the samples in a Microcon-100 column as outlined in *Protocol 3*, steps 11–15.

18. Perform *in vitro* transcription as outlined in *Protocol 4*.

19. You have now generated a second round of aRNA.[b]

[a] This step is done at this stage to remove the RNA in the RNA:cDNA hybrids and to allow the T7 oligo(dT) primer to anneal in step 11.
[b] Quantitate the aRNA using a spectrophotometer. Usually, one needs 5–10 μg aRNA for cDNA probe synthesis to achieve good hybridization signals. If necessary, proceed to a third round.

3.4 Technical considerations of aRNA amplification

There are several important considerations when re-amplifying RNA:

(a) Because the aRNA generated from the initial round is primed with random hexamers, the aRNA obtained after the second round is expected to be slightly shorter in size. For example, one round yields aRNA within a size range of ~ 0.5–3 kb; two rounds yields a size range of ~ 0.4–2.4 kb; and three rounds ~ 0.2–1.5 kb.

(b) When starting with ≥ 1 μg total RNA, one round of amplification is sufficient to generate enough aRNA from which to synthesize fluorescent cDNA probes. Yields are typically 10–20 μg aRNA from 1–2 μg total RNA.

(c) For samples of 10–100 ng total RNA, two rounds of amplification are sufficient; and less than 10 ng of starting material may require three rounds of amplification.

4. cDNA microarrays

4.1 Preparing the cDNAs for the array

With the aid of a Biomek 2000 robot, miniprep DNAs are prepared from bacterial stocks grown in 96-well plates using a Wizard miniprep kit (Promega) according to the manufacturer's protocol. With 5' amino-linked primers, the cDNAs are amplified by PCR using a Perkin Elmer 9600 thermal cycler. The inserts are purified on a Biomek 2000 using Qiagen 96-well PCR purification kit. An aliquot of each amplification reaction is examined on an agarose gel to verify successful amplification. The amplified cDNA inserts are dried down, resuspended in 50 μl 3 × SSC, and stored in 96-well plates at –20°C for printing.

4.2 Preparing the slides

Commercially available silylated slides (CEL Associates) are used as substrates for printing the cDNA PCR products; motion control is accomplished using a custom-made robot. The printing apparatus can accommodate 60 slides per run. On average, spots are about 125 μm in diameter and spacing is 300 μm from centre-to-centre. After printing, the slides are allowed to air dry and are stored at room temperature in slide boxes. Prior to hybridization, the slides are processed according to *Protocol 6*.

Protocol 6. Slide processing

The aldehyde amine chemistry on the slides is a reversible reaction; therefore it is necessary to process the slides with a reducing agent prior to hybridization.

Equipment and reagents
- Sodium borohydrate solution: 0.5 g $NaBH_4$ in 200 ml sterile water plus 4 ml 3 M sodium acetate (pH 5.2)
- 30-slide holder (VWR)

Method

1. Load the slides in a slide holder and soak them in sterile H_2O for 1 min.

2. Soak the slides in sodium borohydrate solution for 5 min.[a]

3. Rinse the slides in H_2O for 1 min.

4. Immerse the slides in boiling water for 2 min.[b]

5. Immerse the slides in 0.2% SDS for 1 min at room temperature.

6. Rinse the slides twice in H_2O for 1 min each at room temperature.

7. Air dry the slides and store them in slide boxes at room temperature.

[a] This step leads to the reduction of the Schiff base that forms between the aldehyde groups on the slide and the amine groups on the DNA.
[b] This step denatures the cDNA on the glass slide.

4.3 Probe synthesis

Protocol 7. Preparation of cDNA probe from aRNA

Equipment and reagents
- Superscript Choice System for cDNA synthesis (Gibco)
- Cy3-dCTP (Amersham)
- Microcon-30 (Millipore)
- Nucleotide removal kit (Qiagen)

Method

1. Combine 5 μg aRNA, 5 μg random hexamers, and DEPC treated water to a total volume of 26 μl.

2. Heat the samples at 70°C for 10 min. Chill the samples on ice.

3. Add 10 μl 5 × first strand buffer, 5 μl 0.1 M DTT, 1.5 μl RNasin, 1 μl 25 mM d(GAT)TP, 2 μl 1 mM dCTP, 2 μl Cy3-dCTP, and 2.5 μl Superscript RT II.

4. Mix the samples gently with a pipette tip and incubate them at room temperature for 10 min.

5. Incubate the reaction at 37°C for 2 h.

6. Add 6 μl 3 M NaOH. Heat the samples at 65°C for 30 min.

7. Add 20 μl 1 M Tris–HCl pH 7.4, 12 μl 1 M HCl, and 12 μl sterile H_2O.

8. Pre-rinse a Microcon-30 column with 500 μl sterile H_2O. Spin the column at 14 000 r.p.m. for 6–7 min in a microcentrifuge.

9. Load each sample in a Microcon-30 column and adjust the volume to 500 μl with sterile H_2O. Spin the samples as in step 8.

10. Purify the probe with Qiagen nucleotide removal column according to the manufacturer's recommended procedure.

11. Recover the probe from the column by eluting in 30 μl sterile H_2O.

4.4 Probe hybridization

Protocol 8. Hybridization/washing

Equipment and reagents
- Perkin Elmer 9600 PCR machine
- Human Cot-1 DNA (Gibco)
- DPX (Fluka)
- Glass coverslips, fine-nosed tweezers, 30-slide holder; glass crystallizing dishes (VWR)
- Hybridization solution: 5 × SSC, 0.2% SDS, 1 mg/ml Cot-1 DNA
- Custom-made hybridization chambers (sealed)

Method

1. Dry down the probe completely after elution from the column (*Protocol 7*, step 11).

2. Resuspend it in hybridization solution. For a 10 mm × 10 mm array, use 5 μl hybridization solution. For an 18 mm × 18 mm array, use 15 μl hybridization solution.

3. Heat the probe solution for 5 min at 99^°C in a Perkin Elmer 9600 PCR machine to prevent evaporation. Cool the probe solution at room temperature for 5 min.

4. Pipette the probe solution just to the side of the array. Place a glass coverslip over the solution and seal the edges with DPX dispensed from a syringe with a 21 gauge needle. Use an 18 mm × 18 mm coverslip for a 10 mm × 10 mm array, and a 22 mm × 30 mm coverslip for an 18 mm × 18 mm array.

5. Hybridize in an airtight hybridization chamber submerged in a 60°C water-bath for 4–6 h.

6. Carefully remove the DPX seal from the glass coverslip and place the slides in a 30-slide holder.[a]

7. Wash the slides once at 55°C in 1 × SSC, 0.2% SDS for 5 min; once in 0.1 × SSC, 0.2% SDS at 55°C for 5 min; and once in 0.1 × SSC at room temperature for 1 min.[b]

8. Spin dry the slides in the rack for a few seconds in a centrifuge that can accommodate 96-well plates.

9. Scan the slides for fluorescence emission.

[a] Note that it is not necessary to remove the glass coverslips because they will fall off easily during wash step 7.
[b] Perform each of these washes with moderate stirring in a glass dish or similar container.

4.5 Scanning and quantitation

After hybridization and washing, each slide was scanned using the ScanArray 3000 (General Scanning, Inc.). Gene expression levels were quantitated using *ImaGene* Software (Biodiscovery, Inc.).

4.6 Microarray experiment

Two sets of neurones (500 and 2500 cells) from rat dorsal root ganglia were laser captured using the PixCell LCM system. The dorsal root ganglia contains different sized neurones (small, medium, and large); in this example, all sizes were captured and pooled. RNA was extracted from each set of cells and checked for integrity by RT–PCR using primers for the rat β-actin and neurone-specific enolase mRNAs. Each RNA preparation was amplified once as outlined in *Protocols 3* and *4* of this chapter and re-amplified twice using *Protocol 5*. A total of three rounds of amplification resulted in about 10^6-fold amplification of the original material.

cDNA probes were synthesized from the aRNA generated from the LCM samples and hybridized to a microarray containing 576 cDNAs. The majority of the cDNAs on the microarray corresponded to genes whose expression was previously identified by differential display to be restricted or enriched in the DRG, as compared to brain, liver, and kidney (18). For negative controls, 30 cDNAs encoding plant genes (gift from M. Schena) were also included in the microarray. The four probes were hybridized to duplicate microarrays, a total of eight arrays were scanned and the data were quantitated.

Figure 3a shows a panel from one of the hybridizations for the 500 cell set and *Figure 3b* shows the same panel on the array from one of the 2500 cell sets. After background correction and normalization of the raw data, each of the duplicate data sets was grouped based on the number of cells used as starting material.

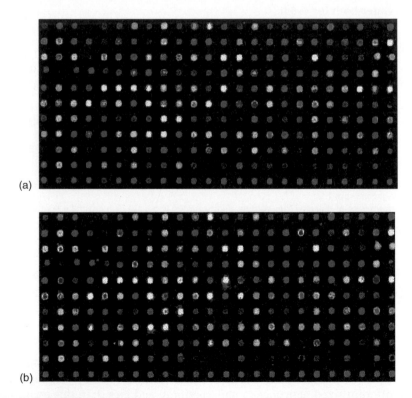

(a)

(b)

Figure 3. Pseudocolour representation of hybridization intensities of cDNA probes synthesized from aRNA amplified from (a) the 500 cell set or (b) the 2500 cell set. Each panel shows the same portion of the array. Pseudocolour intensities: white > violet > blue > green > yellow > orange > red.

The average intensity for each cDNA hybridized with the 500 neurone set (two sets in duplicate or four microarrays), and likewise the average intensity for each cDNA hybridized with the 2500 cell set (four microarrays) were calculated. To determine the reproducibility of the data, we compared the average intensity of four values per cDNA hybridized with either the 500 or the 2500 neurone set. This is graphically represented by plotting them against each other as shown in *Figure 4*. *Table 1* summarizes the sample variation from each data set. Each set had a CV (standard deviation/mean) that was less than 0.2 or 20%.

To further examine reproducibility, we determined the fold-differences between the average hybridization intensity for each cDNA in the 500 cell versus the 2500 cell groups. *Figure 5* shows that the fold-differences between the average measurements derived from the 500 cell groups versus the 2500 cell

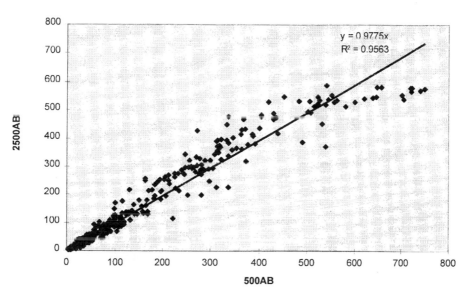

500AB vs 2500AB

$y = 0.9775x$
$R^2 = 0.9563$

Figure 4. Reproducibility between different LCM samples. The average cDNA signal intensity from 2500 neurones versus 500 neurones from rat dorsal root ganglia.

Table 1. Sample variation between duplicate samples

Sample	CV
500 cell set A	18.7%
500 cell set B	15.6%
2500 cell set A	7.8%
2500 cell set B	11.2%

500AB vs 2500AB

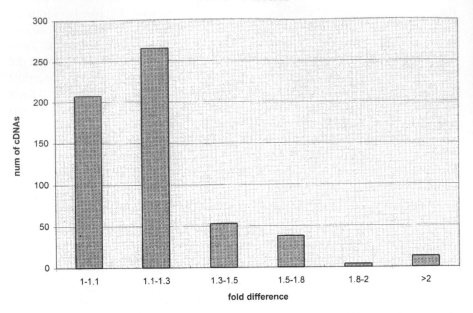

Figure 5. Reproducibility between different LCM samples. Fold-difference between the average measurements for each cDNA in 500 cell versus 2500 cell sets.

groups were in general, relatively small. For example, 472 out of 576 cDNAs or 82% of the cDNAs were only between 1–1.3-fold different; and 97.7% or 563 out of 576 of the cDNAs were less than twofold different. Only 13 out of 576 cDNA intensities or 1.3% were greater than twofold different. These results indicate that different sets of captured cells from the same tissue can yield highly similar results. We have taken this a step further and successfully used LCM, aRNA, and cDNA microarrays to identify differential gene expression between small and large neurones in the dorsal root ganglia. The observed differences in gene expression of individual cDNAs through microarray analysis were subsequently validated by *in situ* hybridization experiments (18).

Acknowledgements

We would like to thank H. Xiao and K. Flores for their assistance in quantitation and K. Witmeyer and V. Le for technical assistance.

References

1. DeRisi, J. L., Iyer, V. R., and Brown, P. O. (1997). *Science*, **278**, 680.
2. Lashkari, D. A., DeRisi, J. L., McCusker, J. H., Namath, A. F., Gentile, C., Hwang, S. Y., *et al.* (1997). *Proc. Natl. Acad. Sci. USA*, **94**, 13057.

3. Schena, M., Shalon, D., Davis, R. W., and Brown, P. O. (1995). *Science*, **270**, 467.
4. Schena, M., Shalon, D., Heller, R., Chai, A., Brown, P. O., and Davis, R. W. (1996). *Proc. Natl. Acad. Sci. USA*, **93**, 10614.
5. DeRisi, J., Penland, L., Brown, P. O., Bittner, M. L., Meltzer, P. S., Ray, M., *et al.* (1996). *Nature Genet.*, **14**, 457.
6. Heller, R. A., Schena, M., Chai, A., Shalon, D., Bedilion, T., Gilmore, J., *et al.* (1997). *Proc. Natl. Acad. Sci. USA*, **94**, 2150.
7. Emmert-Buck, M. R., Bonner, R. F., Smith, P. D., Chuaqui, R. F., Zhuang, Z., Goldstein, S. R., *et al.* (1996). *Science*, **274**, 998.
8. Bonner, R. F., Emmert-Buck, M., Cole, K., Pohida, T., Chuaqui, R., Goldstein, S., *et al.* (1997). *Science*, **278**, 1481.
9. www.arctur.com
10. Sambrook, J., Fritsch, E., and Maniatis, T. (ed.) (1989). *Molecular cloning: a laboratory manual*, 2nd edn. Cold Spring Harbor Laboratory, Cold Spring Harbor, NY.
11. http://dir.niehs.nih.gov/dirlep/lcm.html
12. Krizman, D. B., Chuaqui, R. F., Meltzer, P. S., Trent, J. M., Duray, P. H., Linehan, W. H., *et al.* (1996). *Cancer Res.*, **56**, 5380.
13. Belyavsky, A., Vinogradova, T., and Rajewsky, K. (1989). *Nucleic Acids Res.*, **17**, 2919.
14. Van Gelder, R. N., von Zastrow, M. E., Yool, A., Dement, W. C., Barchas, J. D., and Eberwine, J. H. (1990). *Proc. Natl. Acad. Sci. USA*, **87**, 1663.
15. Eberwine, J., Yeh, H., Miyashiro, K., Cao, X., Nair, S., Finnell, R., *et al.* (1992). *Proc. Natl. Acad. Sci. USA*, **89**, 3010.
16. Poirier, G. M.-C., Pyati, J., Wan, J. S., and Erlander, M. G. (1997). *Nucleic Acids Res.*, **25**, 913.
17. Innis, M. A. and Gelfand, D. H. (1990). In *PCR protocols: a guide to methods and applications* (ed. M. A. Innis, D. H. Gelfand, J. J. Sninsky, and T. J. White), p. 3. Academic Press, San Diego, CA.
18. Luo, L., Salunga, R. C., Guo, H. Q., Bittner, A., Joy, K. C., Galindo, J. E., *et al.* (1999). *Nature Med.*, **5**, 117.

8

Expression data and the bioinformatics challenges

JOEL LLOYD BELLENSON

1. Genes/proteins

1.1 Two aspects of a gene/protein: substance and use values, or sequence/structure and functions

The wealth of those companies and institutions that have embraced genomics or proteomics is represented by the immense accumulation of data regarding genes and proteins. The fundamental unit of wealth being the single gene. Therefore, any presentation of essential bioinformatics must begin with the gene and its intermediate and post-translational products—mRNA and protein.

A gene is a region of DNA that contains the basic template for its transcription into mRNA. This region can be subdivided into other regions or sequences that pertain to coding regions, regulatory regions, and introns. All of these sequences are substantive attributes of the gene which define a large part (but not all) of its ultimate product—the protein.

Sequence analysis has become the cornerstone of bioinformatics because:

(a) Sequence is the primary macromolecular structure data.

(b) It is the most easily obtainable structural data about a molecular function.

From a DNA sequence we can infer a theoretical amino acid sequence. From an amino acid sequence we can infer its secondary structure, and in many cases match it with other protein sequences for which science has already obtained the elusive three-dimensional protein structure. By doing all of the above, we can get as close as we can to knowing the *substance* of the molecular functional unit.

However, just as we know that the substance of charcoal, diamonds, and buckeyballs is fundamentally carbon atoms, and each material has quite different properties, so too knowing the molecular sequence and structure of a gene/protein is insufficient to know its real utility to cellular processes.

Several advanced bioinformatics teams over the years, realizing the limitations of knowing the sequence and structure of single genes and proteins, have attempted to cluster together different genes/proteins that seem to be

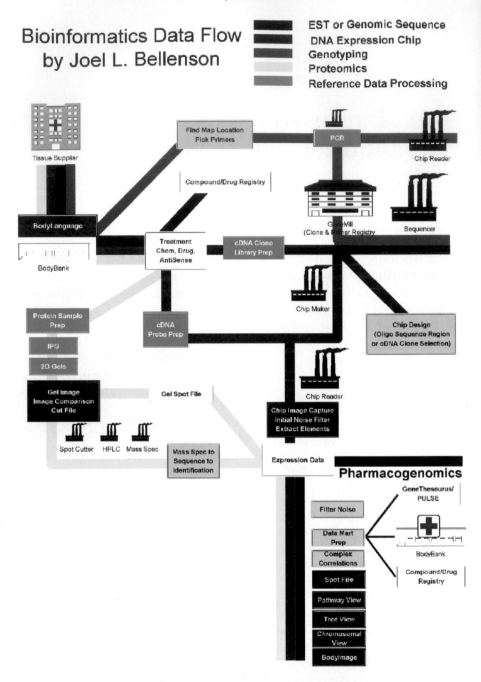

Figure 1. Bioinformatics data flow. The different colours represent some of the principal data types for genomics and proteomics. The interconnections between various data types

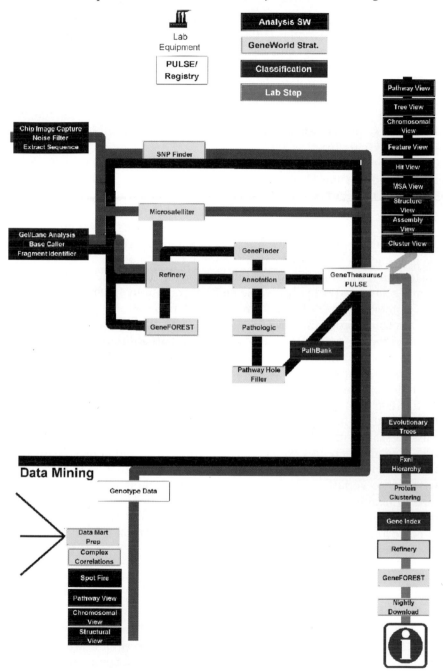

are shown where they intersect at points of utilizing similar sample sources instruments, database references, algorithms, and processes.

evolutionarily related or similar by sequence or structure (1–5). Some of these databases such as Pfam (`http://pfam.wustl.edu/`) are available electronically. In this way, one can leverage whatever spotty, empirical data are available, and try to reason by homology to other genes/proteins within the same cluster or gene/protein family. In effect, these groupings of gene/proteins are attempts at making functional categories. Thus, if we know that this family of proteins is serine kinases, then we can assume that the function of our novel sequence, which seems to match sequences within the family, is also a serine kinase (6).

Other bioinformaticists, faced with the same problem, saw fit to define functional and structural hierarchies. Classification systems such as ENZYME, EGAD, SCOP, CATH (7–10) assign basic biochemical processes, mainly enzymatic function, but others as well, into nested groupings and nominated certain sequences and keywords as representative of that function. Curators of other databases now can use these functional hierarchies to assign novel sequences and attempt to make more sense of their data.

Historically, the study of the association or linkage of the gene sequence variants (genotypes) with observable medical conditions (phenotype) was the most common approach for determining gene function. In the early 90s, its usage was combined with knowledge of crude genetic maps and reoriented to physically locate new genes on chromosomes—positional cloning. The approach was not very fruitful for gene discovery (especially when compared with the expressed sequence tags or ESTs). And in some cases its functional annotations of genes/proteins were superficial and disorienting as they have helped to conceal the real biochemical function of a gene product.

Recently, there has been resurgence in study of gene sequence variation on a massive scale with many genes and large populations of individuals (e.g. SNPs). Unencumbered by the need to discover genes, and in fact, enabled by the resounding success of EST-based gene discovery, there are high hopes that sequence variation will inform us about variations in populations with regard to health, disease, and response to medication. By examining these variations we might learn about the range of a protein's structure/function or how non-protein coding, DNA sequence variation plays a role in altering the timing, conditions, or quantity of gene expression.

1.2 The twofold character of the functions embodied by the gene/protein

1.2.1 Use value and occurrence level, or functions and expression

A worker's physical examination results and job description are not alone indicative of the practical value of a given employee to a company. Similarly, a gene/protein's real utility to a particular cell, in a particular organ, in a particular state of health is not explained by the DNA or protein sequence, the 3D structure, or even the biochemical reaction that it helps to catalyse.

1.2.2 Presence versus absence: an abundance of zeroes

First, and foremost, although every gene is present on its respective chromosome in every cell of an organism, it is not necessarily being transcribed into an active gene product. In fact, the current assumption is that many of the genes are silent or expressed at very low levels in certain cell types. In other words, the number of instances of many genes' mRNA is, presumably zero. So, although we might know exactly what function a gene might code for—its capability or use value—in practice, it might have no utility at all in a particular cell under certain conditions.

Secondly, even when a gene is expressed within a particular cell, its utility is limited by whether or not other genes, that play a vital role in the same cellular process, are present. Thus, to know the utility or relevance of a gene to a given condition, we also need to know about the occurrence level of other genes/proteins involved in the same theoretical molecular pathways. If other genes, essential to the pathway, are not being expressed then the gene/protein in question cannot execute its expected function.

Thirdly, genes are not simple switches to be turned on or off. They are more like thermostats or valves with variable settings. The degree to which a gene is 'turned on' and to which its necessary functional partners are turned on has a quantitative effect on a gene's utility to the cell. Thus the precision of the measurements and the overall bioinformatics system, impact all other downstream calculations.

1.3 Relative and absolute occurrence levels: constrained by our methods

The amount of a particular gene that is objectively present in a particular sample is simultaneously an absolute measurement and a relative measurement. None the less, since our current techniques cannot identify and measure every mRNA molecule in a sample, we end up with only a relative occurrence value. We know the ratio of the number of copies of a particular mRNA to the total number of mRNAs collected and identified. This is the case whether we are sequencing ESTs or hybridizing cDNA libraries to microarrays. The absence of a reliable absolute occurrence value lies at the root of many problems associated with doing comparisons between physiological samples.

One of the most common problems resulting from the measuring of relative occurrence is that the overall uniqueness of the cell or tissue or disease state we are measuring is contributing to the differential skewing of the relative occurrence of the particular gene(s) we might be looking at. In other words, the overall effect of the different levels of many genes can have a serious impact on the relative occurrence of a few genes. This is an effect that is not as significant for genes with high absolute copy numbers, but is very damaging for the analysis of lower copy number genes wherein small changes in ratio might be significant biochemically. In fact, because other molecules may be present in such large relative amounts, we might get the false impression that the gene(s) of interest are not present. Thus, our lack of true absolute occurrence measurements puts us in a situation where we cannot believe in the value of zero. This turns out to have a number of repercussions for comparative data analysis and the understanding of molecular function.

If values of zero cannot be relied upon to be truly zero, then the earlier question of presence versus absence can only be answered with some degree of uncertainty. Can that uncertainty be quantified as a confidence level? Possibly, after exhaustive focused experimentation on numerous cell types, confidence levels for the absences of various genes could be established.

Since zero cannot be relied upon, the value of one might be questionable, since it too could be artificially low due to sampling error. Establishing standard deviations for normal expression levels for various genes would be immensely helpful.

To obviate these problems many researchers have resorted to creating 'normalized' libraries wherein commonly occurring, highly abundant genes, 'housekeeping genes', are filtered away leaving a mixture of transcripts enriched for the lower copy number genes. This approach allows greater confidence in a zero value, but it might be skewing the gene occurrence ratios when two samples are compared since they may have differing amounts of 'housekeeping genes'. Utilization of the absolute gene occurrence values must be done with full knowledge of the *total mRNA level before normalization* so that a relative gene occurrence value can be generated for comparison purposes.

Another approach is to create 'subtracted' libraries wherein pairs of samples are treated such that only the mRNAs in sample A and not in sample B, or vice versa, remain to be hybridized or sequenced. This approach promises better absolute numbers for each sample, more visibility into the low copy gene zone, and a clean comparison between the two samples. None the less, the resulting data is limited in its usefulness for global comparisons to other samples. The values can only be usefully compared when a gene is present in both samples, otherwise the gene's absence can be explained as a result of the laboratory subtraction instead of as a real absence in the sample.

1.4 The fetishism of genes/proteins

The function of a gene/protein appears at first to be a fairly straightforward thing. It is a 'kinase', or an 'ion channel', or a 'receptor', or 'neurotransmitter'. But on further inspection we find that understanding gene/protein function becomes very complex and tentative and almost mysterious.

Because current technologies for quantifying the presence of a particular functional unit let us do it for a multitude of genes simultaneously, they enable us to think about function at a whole, new level—that of networks of interactions between molecules within biochemical pathways.

Once this higher level of thought is entered into, the radical inadequacy of the other becomes apparent. Fixation on the function of a single gene/protein in isolation from the associated actors in the cell is understandable only as an experimental approach but not as scientific method because:

(a) A gene is not a protein and therefore has no function of its own.

(b) A single gene does not code for a single protein; alternate splicing of mRNA and post-translational modification leads to a one-to-many relationship.

(c) Protein level and activity is not the result of a single gene. Promoters and inhibitors govern its expression level. Proteolytic cleavage, phosphorylation, and glycosylation uniquely and materially alter the raw translated protein. These processes involve numerous other gene products.

(d) A single protein does not always have a single biochemical function or cellular role.

(e) Proteins exert their influence or function *by acting in concert* with one another and with other molecules, including hormones, metabolites, and yes, regulatory regions of DNA.

None the less, we are faced with some huge difficulties to overcome if we are to perform a holistic analysis and move away from the single gene/protein fetish. In fact, only when faced with the frustratingly close-at-hand holistic

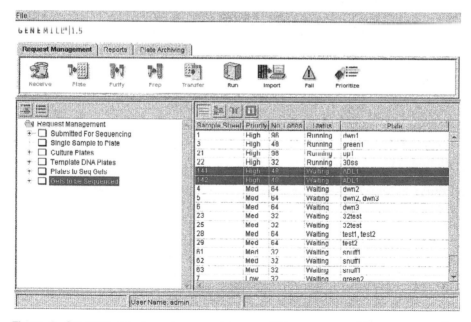

Figure 2. GeneMill sample management screen. This screen provides a commanding console to manage the massive, rapid, and complex flows of data from automated DNA sequencing instruments.

analysis do we finally understand why molecular science had seemingly stalled out at the single gene fixation level. Our notion of function is fundamentally rooted in:

(a) The sensitivity of our laboratory methods.

(b) Our ability to co-ordinate, organize, process, pre-digest, and visualize all of the related reference data about every gene/protein.

Those data, whether it be sequence or structure or map location, empirically observed biochemical function, known chemical inhibitors, algorithmically predicted attributes, and the entire network of known or predicted interactions between molecules must all be accessible within a common information management and software development environment. To the extent to which this is not the case, the function of a molecule, and the basic biochemistry of life, will continue to be obscured.

The next sections lay out the basic elements of the bioinformatics logistics and decision support infrastructures necessary to get the most value from expression data.

2. The raw data pipeline

2.1 Libraries, clones, sequences, and EST clusters

The most mundane and often overlooked component of the system is that of the physical sample management (*Figure 1*). One could easily argue that this omission is behind the atrocious reproducibility levels of all the major sequencing houses. Clones ordered from these institutions based on interest in the reported sequence, upon arrival and re-sequencing match the reported sequence less than 50% of the time.

Such a system can be highly interactive, whereby the technicians are frequently noting the passage of each sample through each stage of its preparation in the laboratory on its way toward becoming a sequencing run on an instrument (*Figure 2*). For large scale, well-automated laboratories that handle samples in large batches (e.g. 96- or 384-well or bigger plates), the level of interaction cannot be upon the sample and must be upon the plate. In fact, in some laboratories the preference is for the robots themselves to be automatically interacting with the database workflow system through their bar code readers and the database's application programming interface (API).

Sequence data derived from the clones and physiological samples is inherently associated through the structure of the database. This allows a higher fidelity of clone sequence matching which is essential for other usages of the clones downstream such as full-length sequencing or the gridding of cDNA onto microarrays.

Sequences can then be automatically passed on to algorithmic strategies (*Figure 3*), which make use of various bioinformatics tools to improve on the quality of the data. Typically, ESTs need to have the artefacts of the molecular biology techniques that produced them removed: poly(A) tails, vector sequence. In addition, other sequences need to be deleted from the project. These include those bacterial as well as mitochondrial sequences. Finally, repetitive elements must be identified and masked so that they do not cause spurious matches to one another.

Since one of the goals of expression analysis is to get quantitative information, when using ESTs we have to go through a major data reduction process. This process fundamentally is concerned with clustering ESTs into groups of overlapping sequences that match in their overlapping regions with extremely high fidelity. Once these groupings are generated, the group memberships and totals can be stored in the database and related back to the physiological samples. These totals then become the raw abundance numbers that, when divided by the total number of sequences surveyed in a physiological sample, provide the relative abundance level of a particular gene.

Bioinformaticists have used a number of techniques to accomplish this using typical homology search algorithms such as *BLAST*, *FASTA*, and *Smith-Waterman* (11–13). In some cases, they would search every EST against a database using one of these algorithms and then group together those query sequences that matched the same sequence in the reference database. This was reasonable for known genes, but not very helpful for the unknowns. In other laboratories, they would make a large database of all ESTs available to them and do a search of all against all. This got around the problem of not being able to group together unknown sequences. However, it has become intolerably slow, especially as the databases of ESTs have grown in both the public and private domain. In addition, these clustering methods have significant problems with chimeras, contamination, poor data curation, and cannot provide any insights into alternate mRNA splice forms (*Figure 4*).

Burke *et al.* (Pangea Systems, Inc.) have developed a method of clustering ESTs that is extremely rapid, scalable, accurate, and sensitive (14). The throughput of this approach on a standard, single processor, desktop workstation is approximately one million ESTs per day! It can be scaled with multiple processors and more RAM. The method weeds out chimeras, contamination, and corrects for wrong orientated sequences. In addition, it performs subcluster analysis and can therefore identify isogenes—alternative mRNA splice forms. Pangea has made the tools available and licensed them to several pharmaceutical companies who have invested heavily in EST-based expression analysis.

2.2 Microarray data

2.2.1 Gene selection and chip design

Much has been written about the capabilities of DNA chips to analyse thousands of genes in parallel. Even though these chips represent a major breakthrough, they still do not allow the scientist to abdicate responsibility for creating a more limited experiment. In short, the chips do not have sufficient density to simultaneously monitor with high precision the occurrence level of every gene. Furthermore, once gene isoforms and other sequence variants are considered for purposes of expression, it becomes clear that the chips would have to become much more densely gridded before the question of gene selection is rendered obsolete.

The process of gene selection is one that goes through automated analysis, sequence homology, and database queries. Using standard algorithms combined with the reference data warehouse (discussed below) users can make subsets of genes that they wish to have gridded onto a chip.

Unfortunately, once the genes are selected, the work gets very difficult and tedious. Since the sequences in the databases are not all correctly oriented and there are a variety of problems with sequencing artefacts and repetitive elements, merely getting the right sequences together is a chore. Furthermore, many genes are very similar. As noted above, genes and proteins can be grouped into various families within which sequences are fairly similar. Since the user wants to make a quantitative determination of occurrence level of different, unique genes, it is desirable to select characteristic regions of the gene sequences; these afford the ability to discriminate between otherwise very similar genes.

Culling through the databases including the EST repositories and putting together optimal contigs, selecting appropriately characteristic regions of uniqueness, and determining the layout of these sequences onto a chip are not easy tasks. It can take a skilled bioinformaticist a few months to design a single chip. However, Burke *et al.* (Pangea Systems, Inc.) have devised an automated system for chip design that enables rapid determination of appropriate regions for chip layout.

2.2.2 Images, numbers, and genes

Regardless of the technology involved in creating the microarray, the data types involved are basically the same. Whether the chip is based on using oligonucleotides or amplified cDNA fragments, the resulting data from most current detection systems are initially an image that has captured the intensities at various wavelengths of emitted fluorescent light. The various hardware vendors have each written their own software for image capture. In the case of the Genetics Analysis Technology Consortium (GATC), which so far includes Affymetrix and Molecular Dynamics (now owned by Amersham/ Pharmacia), they have devised and published a normalized database schema that allows the description of various experimental parameters involved in the cDNA probe preparation, hybridization, detection, and deconvolution process. Although each has written their own applications on top of this schema, their intent was to provide a common repository for the raw microarray data regardless of whether it came from an oligonucleotide-based or an amplified cDNA fragment-based source.

(Note: there are several other major companies competing in this space which have not joined the GATC, notably Incyte/Synteni, Hyseq, and Perkin Elmer Biosystems. In fact, they have their own software that operates on their own proprietary schemas. Such software as Incyte/Synteni's *GEMTools* and *LifeArray* is available for looking at the raw image data and performing simple comparison operations on expression profiles. In addition, there are over a dozen other companies offering low to medium density arrays for expression analysis that may or may not have any software for interpreting their raw image data.)

Assuming that one does have a vendor who has software for interpreting the microarray images, one is left with a large pile of numbers of various precision and meaning in a database. So the task ahead is to link that raw numeric data back to:

(a) The gene/protein sequence/structure/functional data.

(b) The medical/physiological/demographic information associated with the sample being studied.

However, this task of linkage is severely constrained if the necessary data are not being aggregated and readily available for use. The following sections explain the 'why' and the 'what' of data aggregation.

3. The reference data warehouse

3.1 Why warehouse?

To the naive researcher, it might appear to be a trivial task to find information related to a given gene/protein. After all, the web is littered with databases and most desktop sequence analysis packages have a sequence database and maybe even a database of 3D coordinates for the protein structure. So what's the problem? In fact, given that all of these databases are constantly changing, why wouldn't one just want to link up to them where they were, on an as-needed basis?

Linking to a loose federation of databases would be fine for performing simple look-ups, assuming the net connections were stable and not slowed unduly by everyone else's multimedia surfing. And it would be fine if you did not mind sending your private sequence information out over unencrypted lines. However, the situation is substantially different when you want to do sophisticated, real time, data mining behind the security of your company's firewall or at least a secure connection.

To structure the data so that complex queries and algorithms can work on huge disparate databases requires a robust, integrative architecture and flexible, intelligent, automated processes to churn through millions of records in a variety of incompatible formats.

Here are ten imperatives, that drive the bioinformatics reference data warehouse.

(a) The relevant data must be collated. This will mean somehow getting the appropriate licensing arrangements and then downloading the databases.

(b) The databases have important cross-references to one another, that can be leveraged to build a more comprehensive view of the data about a gene/protein.

(c) The data in the databases is often semi-overlapping, inconsistent, and often derivative of yet another database.

(d) Each database has its own data structure or format, which in addition, is unstable and inconsistent.

(e) Each database has its own rhythm to the timing of its release dates; thus there never is a convenient time of the month or year to declare all information up-to-date.

(f) Some databases are subscriptions to proprietary collections; these have their own restrictions on usage or royalties associated.

(g) Internal researchers are always augmenting existing data with new observations of their own; these sometimes extend and other times conflict with existing information.

(h) Bioinformaticists can utilize powerful algorithms to compare data and extend the relevance of sparse observational data thus producing databases of computational or predictive content.

(i) Companies and universities are often in collaboration involving other institutions and therefore the sharing of data between them becomes crucial while the need for proprietary control still remains.

(j) Issues of sharing or publishing and privacy exist also within every institution as individuals and projects want to hold onto their data until they have verified it; at which point, they want to publish it to a wider internal corporate community. From the information administration perspective, new, automation-driven discoveries need to be disseminated throughout the organization to those whose specialities are involved. For example, an algorithm finds a remote homology match of a previously unknown sequence to a protein family for which someone is an expert at modelling protein structure and rational drug design.

4. The structure of molecular information

4.1 Sequence, structure, function, and other attributes

No other type of biological information has received as much attention as DNA sequences. Partly because they define the essence of what has been molecular biology and partly because it used to be a daunting challenge to store such large chunks of information, sequence data banks have been designed, and probably over designed, many times over.

As a result, a few main points can be firmly concluded:

(a) A particular gene sequence is only one instance of a gene.

(b) There is no ideal sequence that exists in nature.

(c) Every gene has many partial sequences associated with it.

(d) Numerous intervals along a gene sequence can be defined and associated with other information.

(e) A gene sequence itself occupies an interval along a chromosomal sequence.

Similar points can be made about a protein's sequence and three-dimensional structure. The main point of departure being that a protein sequence is not part of a larger sequence, although it is an active part of a larger molecular environment including complexes of proteins.

Biochemical function lurks haphazardly in most sequence databases. Sometimes systematically located in the same slot, but rarely described systematically. With wide ranging vocabulary, poor spelling, and often virtually vacuous meaning, the precious nuggets of knowledge about function are denigrated. One might hunt for the function of a gene within a single database looking at record titles, descriptions, keywords, and sequence features. Grammar and context are not always clear. Nouns and adjectives are used interchangeably. Subject is confused with object. Genes and their corresponding proteins have numerous aliases with confusing cross-references. It is a persistent problem, whose manifestations are not consistent.

The scientific community is starting to cry out in pain and alarm at the collective and synergistic inadequacy of the numerous and expensive attempts to catalogue molecular function.

4.2 Singular and plural

If science is to avoid drowning in unfathomable data, molecular biologists must come to terms with some very basic facts, which seem to get acknowledged in one breath and denied by every other:

(a) A gene is not a protein and therefore has no function of its own.

(b) A single gene does not code for a single protein (alternative splicing, post-translational modification).

(c) A protein is not a product of a single gene.

(d) A single ideal gene sequence does not exist.

(e) A single protein does not always have a single biochemical function or cellular role.

(f) Proteins exert their influence or function *by acting in concert* with one another and with other molecules, including hormones, metabolites, and yes, regulatory regions of DNA.

In short, there must be a conceptual leap that can accommodate the plurality contained within the unity, and that the unity itself is a part of a multiplicity at a higher level and therefore contained within another unity. Proteins exist within cells, which exist within an individual organism, which exists within a population, which are part of an ecosystem. There must be no confusion between the usage of reductionist methods of study and the fact that the ultimate thing being studied exists in a higher level of organization that is much richer than the sum of its reduced parts.

4.3 Universal versus situational

When functional observations are made, much more care needs to be taken to accommodate the richness of the context of the observation. Databases are filled with keywords and descriptions about genes/proteins; these have the appearance of universal truth and applicability. The march of time will eventually accumulate enough contradictions with the original observation so that we will realize its limitations; however, why not take careful note of (i.e. store in the database) for example, whether or not the experiment was *in vivo*, *in vitro*, or in silico? What cell type or subcellular fraction was analysed? Which stage of development the experimental subject is passing through?

The greater the detail that can be noted and stored the better the data mining that can be performed later. Although this will mean the accumulation of much redundant data or a sparsely filled column, digital storage space is no longer at such a premium that it can be allowed to truncate the tracking of the conditions of the observations.

4.4 Degrees of knowledge: uncertain, unknown, unimportant

Commentators on molecular and cellular biology and evolution are polarizing into two great camps. One holds to the reductionist, gene centred or mechanical materialist view a la Richard Dawkins in *The Selfish Gene* (15); the other abandons material explanations and turns to divine design a la Michael Behe in Darwin's Black Box (16). Either view is disastrous if put in command of structuring bioinformatics data.

The narrow, gene fetishist, mechanical materialist cannot cope with the subjectivity, multiplicity, interdependence, complexity, and conditionality of the functional observations and therefore will ignore the need to constantly, and iteratively, track the often declining level of confidence in a particular finding.

The believer in divine design inherently confuses the unknown with the unknowable; and they confuse both with the unimportant. S/he will therefore fail to either define the properties that are still unknown or acknowledge and update the information once it has been acquired. Worse yet, since their a priori conclusion is that the biochemistry of life is basically well designed, they will tend to ignore observations of functional redundancy, secondary functions, contradictory functions, and historical development.

Finally, the thorniest problem is when to acknowledge that some attribute is irrelevant or not applicable. One can say with confidence that the pK_a of a gene does not exist or that the attributes of GC content or promoter region are not applicable to a protein.

For the empirical researcher, these types of questions form the boundaries of their observations and are settled up-front. However, for the information management system designer and administrator, this is an ongoing struggle. New technologies are constantly emerging that provide opportunities to detect types of data previously hidden or improve the certainty or sensitivity of data already obtained. The question of whether this new data type applies to other cases is relevant to whether the database gets populated with zeroes, 'null', or 'does not apply'. The values that get inserted into the database then determine whether that information can be used in graphs, charts, statistical calculations, algorithms, heuristics, pattern matching, and rule detection.

4.5 The coming transitive catastrophe: observations, inferences, references, and subscriptions

Much of the data contained in bioinformatics databases about genes and proteins is derivative. In fact, aside from the raw sequence data which itself is the result of a submission from a third party, most of the data in GenBank, Swiss-Prot, and especially the numerous smaller databases is either based upon information stored somewhere else or has been calculated on top of some other data source.

Some examples:

(a) The protein sequence in SwissProt is the result of translating the DNA sequences in GenBank or EMBL into an amino acid sequence using the appropriate codon translation table for that species.

(b) Database cross-references are often the result of applying sequence comparison algorithms.

(c) Sequence features are often the result of using multiple sequence alignment tools.

(d) Full-length sequences or at least the longest possible contigs are derived from EST data through clustering algorithms.

(e) Gene sequences are located within larger genomic sequences through the use of gene finding or ORF finding algorithms.

(f) Protein structures are assigned to sequences through sequence homology and threading.

While incredibly sophisticated computational approaches have provided enormous leverage of sparse biological data, the community's immaturity at

Joel Lloyd Bellenson

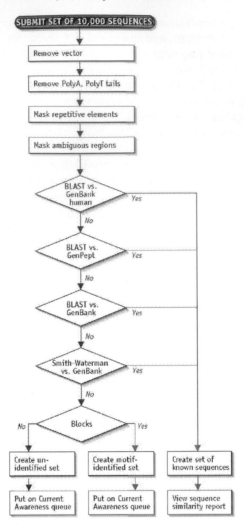

Figure 3. GeneWorld strategy. This flow chart depicts a bioinformatics approach to analysis of a large set of sequences for purposes of annotation and functional analysis. The flow chart represents the capture of logic that can then be systematically and automatically applied to a collection of data.

database management and information modelling has built several skyscrapers of cards. Since so many databases are interdependent, real changes to underlying data has a massive ripple effect on every other database. Since Database A refers to Database B which refers to Database C, A relies on C. This has been transitive leverage, but it is perched on the edge of catastrophe.

The pace of these updates will only grow as high-throughput techniques are applied to elucidating DNA sequence variation and protein function. Of course, current systems do not even handle gene expression data in any sophisticated way let alone protein expression data, protein–protein inter-action data, or chemical screening data.

The problem cries out for powerful architecture, however most scientists are oblivious to the problem and illiterate to the possible information man-agement solutions. Since very few bioinformatics experts are database experts and since every industry is devouring data management expertise, the prob-lem has received scant attention.

Fortunately, some scientists have seen this problem coming for awhile and have been building a system—GeneWorld/GeneThesaurus with the robustness and human programmable strategies that might avert the looming catastrophe.

Any architecture that attempts to address the enormity of the challenge, will have to be able to:

(a) Distinguish between genuine observations and inferences made by soft-ware or people.

(b) Track in detail every reference a database makes to another database, including all the points made above concerning confidence levels and whether something is knowable or relevant or current.

(c) Track who relies upon it. Just as someone who is diagnosed with AIDS should be able to notify their former partners that they are at risk, so should a database be able to notify its subscribers when data has become revealed to be incorrect.

(d) Reproduce the usage of the various algorithms in the appropriate sequence with the appropriate conditional logic which generated the derivative data after an update.

5. Medical lexicon and donor sample registration

The analysis of gene and protein expression data requires not only the attach-ment of quantitative measurements with the plethora of molecular informa-tion, but also a structured approach to describing the physiological samples that are being analysed. Most systems in use provide cursory descriptions of the medical conditions of the individual or sample being analysed. These have been largely unstructured textual details culled from pathology reports pro-vided by the tissue supplier. This approach inhibits the systematic analysis of the data using medical descriptors.

The principal problem is that every clinician uses slightly different termin-ology for similar conditions. This can prevent the aggregating of multiple samples together that really should be grouped by disease state or demo-graphic information or part of the body.

Fortunately there are several systems for codifying medical terminology. These systems were developed to answer the similar needs of hospitals,

Joel Lloyd Bellenson

ALIGNMENT CONTAINS INCONSISTENCY:Strong Secondary Consensus Found.

One position equals 33 bases.
■ if more than 3 bases (10 percent) disagree with consensus sequences.
■ if more than 3 positions are unknown.
_ if more than 16 positions are gap characters.

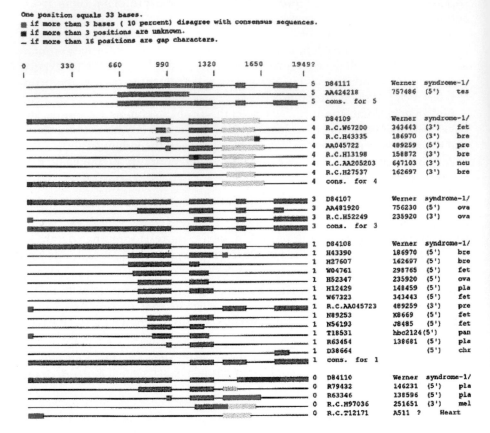

Figure 4. CRAW viewer of gene isoforms. An alignment of EST is displayed that shows the subclusters within a cluster. These subclusters represent alternative splice forms that demonstrate tissue and disease specificity in their expression.

research institutions, health maintenance organizations, insurance companies, pathology laboratories, and diagnostic clinics. The most commonly used coding systems are SNOMED, ICD, CPT, MediSpan (17–20). These overlap with one another but roughly correspond to pathology, diagnoses, surgical procedures, and current medications. These coding systems are semi-overlapping and have deficiencies in the level of detail in some cases and in extreme verbosity in others.

Pangea Systems, Inc. has exclusively licensed a curated, interlinked lexicon from Intelligent Medical Objects and is tailoring it for use in genomic and proteomic analysis. Such a lexicon enables the rapid, accurate, and systematic registration of donor and sample information from existing medical paperwork about a sample. Having the information systematically structured, unlike a textual description, facilitates database searching and the use of various pattern matching and other heuristics and algorithms in the data mining phase of analysis.

6. Data mining an expression data mart

6.1 Analytical versus transactional systems of data management

Most of the modern database design approaches arose in response to rapidly acquire data from numerous transactions, wherein various pieces of information in somewhat separate systems needed to be consulted or updated before a transaction was completed. The most typical example of this is in the financial services sector where various accounts are constantly being updated through the actions of individual users as well as automatic calculations made on the account activities within various market places. These systems had to be designed to be extremely fast at performing atomized actions; and the system had to be accurate up to the second. For that reason, database designers build transactional systems primarily in a way that corresponds to storing data in the least possible redundant manner. This optimizes the existence of information already within the system during basic data entry by ensuring the integrity of the data since fundamental information is only entered once and is subjected to the business rules encapsulated in the database application software code. None the less, the same features that make these on-line transaction processing systems (OLTP) very fast, efficient, and accurate, also make them very difficult to query.

There has been a trend in the last five years towards what is called on-line analytical processing (OLAP). These systems are designed to take the data acquired through the various OLTP systems that a company may have and reorganize into a fashion that allows easier and faster querying of current information. These systems, to achieve their speed benchmarks, employ two main approaches. First, the conscious creation of highly redundant information that reduces the need to look at numerous database tables to answer a query. Secondly, the utilization of new technologies for indexing and caching the data. In both approaches, the common theme is that the nature of the questions drive how the data get organized. In OLTP, the fundamental structure of the information drove the design of the database schema, in OLAP the reports drive the schema. For such an approach to be highly successful, requires systematically analysing the types of questions that the users need the system to answer. Then the data can be subjected to pre-processing approaches so that it is constructed in a fashion that facilitates those defined query approaches. These pre-processing approaches must be automatic and triggered by significant updates in the underlying data coming through the OLTP systems that feed into the OLAP systems.

In the case of molecular expression analysis, think of GenBank, SwissProt (21, 22), and the other canonical bioinformatics databases as OLTP systems. Next think of the sequence/function reference data warehouse and processing engine as an intermediate, hybrid, conglomerated OLTP system with some OLAP restructuring for fast and easy querying of sequence/structure/function related questions. Think of the laboratory sample tracking, sequence data harvesting, chip data harvesting, or 2D proteomics gel/mass spec data harvesting systems all as pure OLTP. Finally, think of the expression data mart as one of the resulting by-product OLAP systems dedicated to the synthesis of the quantitative information from clustered ESTs, DNA chips, or protein gel/mass spec with the physiological sample registration system, chemical/medicinal registration systems, and the molecular reference data.

6.2 In silico hypothesis testing and hypothesis discovery

The hypothesis is the cornerstone of scientific research and the evaluation or formulation of a hypothesis with empirical data is nothing new. However, what is new is the sheer magnitude of the data. Whereas before, various associations might have been made by the scientist with the revered memorization capabilities who could cross-correlate various attributes in her/his head. The scale of the data now makes the success of this type of natural brilliance ever more rare. For this reason, scientists turn to using computational models, simulations, clustering approaches, neural networks, machine-based learning approaches, and pattern recognition systems to either:

(a) Suggest a possible correlation or hypothesis.

(b) Test out the universality of a new hypothesis against different sets of data.

While in both modes—hypothesis discovery and hypothesis testing—the scientist is using software with data to get insights or rule out possible explanations, these are two different phases of the scientific process (although they interpenetrate with one another). The difference between these two phases is what drives the selection or, more likely today, the design of the appropriate software tools.

6.3 Analysis tools: algorithms and heuristics

The world of bioinformatics tools has devoted itself almost exclusively to the development of algorithms and rules for handling DNA and protein sequences. With the advent of copious amounts of expression data tied in with molecular, medical, and chemical data bioinformaticists have a new challenge: to develop tools that enable the systematic analysis of molecular expression.

Much earlier software effort was focused on performing standard set manipulations such as 'electronic subtractions'. These operations pointed out what genes were strongly up- or down-regulated. They also enabled the identification of genes that were expressed in common between tissues of varying disease states and therapeutic approaches. Electronic Northerns provided the ability to note the changes of a select number of genes across disease states or time points, or across various physiological systems, or of various dosages of treatments versus untreated patients.

Researchers have begun employing basic statistical approaches for finding quantitatively correlated genes or 'gene cliques'. The real power of such statistical correlation approaches will come from bringing in various types of annotation information from the reference databases. For example, by including chromosomal location or biochemical pathway information or protein structural classification into the data marts which the statistical algorithms will process, it might be possible to detect correlations not just of a purely numeric kind, but rather with real biological context.

The more biological information included with the expression data marts, the more opportunities to develop better algorithms whose results could be validated against the reference data and expected behaviour. In addition, as the algorithms mature they will incorporate various rules of thumb that biologists already intuitively know. These rules of thumb will help the algorithms' sensitivity, accuracy, and usefulness substantially. For example, by identifying a gene as coding for a transcription factor, when the algorithmic logic is processing through expression values, the fact that a transcription factor is expressed in very low quantities will not preclude seeing an association with the expression of another gene and its pathway. Without that heuristic, a key linkage between several genes would be invisible and discounted by the uninformed algorithm. These heuristics will be numerous and immensely valuable. They will embody a lot of existing knowledge, but will also need to be grown out of what is learned from the new large scale data sources.

6.4 Visualization of data versus visualization of information

For many scientists, the software for visualization is all that matters. Since visualization is synonymous with the asking or answering of questions, this point of view is appropriate regardless of the Herculean tasks necessary to agglomerate, collate, normalize, pre-process the underlying data. (Those who have skipped the bulk of this chapter just to read this section should go back and absorb some of the earlier points in light of how they might impact on visualization. Think especially about questions of uncertainty, the usage of zero, null, and irrelevance, and valuations for multifunctional proteins.)

6.5 The genomic parts list and the chip data as bill of material

The microarray- and EST-based expression data provide science with a type and amount of data that cries out for new approaches to visualization (*Figure 5*). The basic form of visualization has been a list, whether of differentially

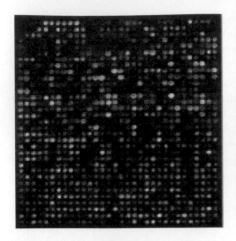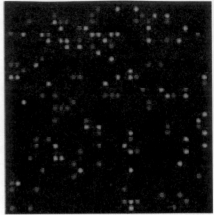

Figure 5. Chip images. The colours represent various intensities of expression of thousands of genes. Although very pretty to look at, the biological implications remain hidden in such a view. The main utility is for laboratory technicians who operate the instruments for creation, hybridization, and imaging of chips. Using such an image is valuable for detecting and troubleshooting problems in the laboratory process.

expressed genes (transcript profile) or of quantities of the same gene expressed in differing contexts (Northern). The list is the basis of visualization of genes on a chromosome or of the sequence motifs on a gene. In fact, one can say that fundamentally, the entire goal of the human genome project has been to get The List—whether sequentially ordered by mapping information or willy-nilly collected and clustered from ESTs.

Now when confronted with quantitative information about some of the items on The List another list is made, and this is the transcript or expression profile or chip image. It is a smaller list but it has a number next to it. This number is either a ratio between two contexts or merely the number for a single experimental context. It is still a list; and it can be ordered by quantity or alphabetically or functional categorically, but it is a list and it is manifestly limiting to one's ability to form and test hypothesis.

6.6 Graphing/mathematics packages

Certainly there is substantial benefit in using these lists with traditional tools for graphing data whether in 2D or 3D axis graphs. Many biopharmaceutical firms make use of *Excel*, *SAS*, *SigmaGraph*, or *Cricket Graph*, and there are new tools within the same genre such as *SpotFire*, *CrossGraph*, or *MineSet*, which try to look at expression data in a more exploratory sense.

SpotFire and *CrossGraphs* provide highly configurable 2D views of the data and allow the utilization of the systems of classification that have been indexed into the expression data mart. *MineSet* is bundled with Incyte's *LifeSeq* and provides eye-candy with a video game-like flyover of functional hierarchies graphed quantitatively.

The above methods do provide some utility especially when one is zeroing in on a small number of genes whose expression levels are being monitored. However, if one wants to look at broader effects throughout the cell or body, lists and axes on graphs are not very helpful.

6.7 Organic information structures

Although our knowledge of biology is still very limited it can be organized and visualized according to whatever paradigms are helpful.

6.7.1 Example 1: evolutionary trees

Although the regulatory mechanisms and map locations of all the genes are largely unknown, one can still organize proteins according to their evolution- ary tree relationships within a protein superfamily. Once that is done, expres- sion data can be painted onto the tree (*Figure 6*) and then one can clearly see which genes are being expressed together in particular tissue or disease contexts (23).

Because the proteins are already subclustered and those subclusters seem to match fairly well with expression localization, one might be able to make or break initial hypotheses about regulatory processes. And given that many drugs are designed to target a small collection of target structure archetypes (approx. 40 superfamilies representing 400 different proteins), being able to see expression in the context of the subclustering within a superfamily can be very helpful in ascertaining localization effects and general tendencies toward co-expression.

6.7.2 Example 2: pathway diagrams

There is substantial literature about molecular mechanisms and biochemical pathways. Some of that has been organized into metabolic pathway databases, most notably EcoCyc (24), but also KEGG (25), and WIT (26). And now that EcoCyc has been privatized, Pangea Systems, Inc. has made it the largest database of pathways in the world, including many signalling and transport pathways.

More than being a reference look-up system of well-curated data on par- ticular organisms, it is a system for the registration and visualization of path- ways. Because it can make use of any other data in the entire data warehouse or data mart it can paint quantitative expression data from DNA chips or 2D proteomic gels directly onto complex pathway overview diagrams (*Figure 7*).

This is a revolutionary capability for it converts the genomics parts list or the expression bill of materials into a real schematic of cellular function. When one looks at the data in its true biological context, meaning can jump right out instead of having to scour lists and axes hoping to find something to leap out by name or by number. Pathway diagrams are one of the fundamental

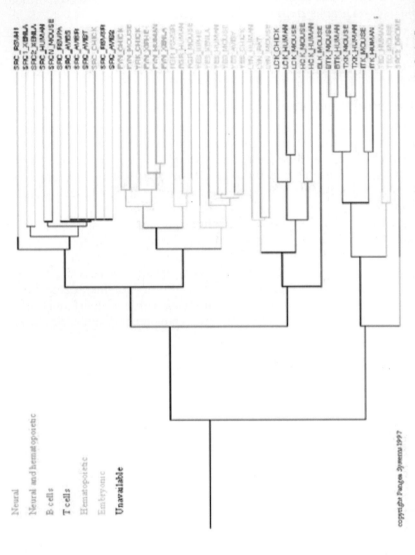

Figure 6. Evolutionary trees with expression painted on. An evolutionary tree built from protein sequences in SwissProt to depict the evolutionary distances between sequences containing SH2 domains. Overlaid onto the tree are coloured subclusters representing localization of expression in various physiological systems and cell types.

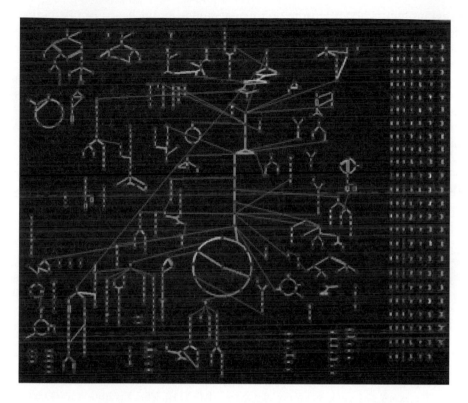

Figure 7. Pathway diagram with expression painted on. This is a metabolic (and signalling) pathway diagram depicting molecular interactions that occur in yeast. The automatic coloration is derived from Affymetrix DNA chip data and represents the degree and direction of relative expression between two samples of yeast, one starved and then later fed.

methods of understanding biochemistry; and expression data whether from ESTs, microarrays, or proteomic gels/mass spec or chips are fundamentally quantitative assays for the presence of various biochemicals in the cell. No other method of visualization can provide as much cellular context, speed up knowledge acquisition, and acclimate the newly initiated project member or collaborator as a pathway diagram combined with expression data.

7. Conclusion

Despite the enormous technical advances in speed, precision, and sensitivity on the laboratory instrumentation, we are still in the infancy of our knowledge of molecular and cellular physiology and function. Only now have we been forcefully presented with a sufficient quantity and type of data so that previous hubris about information management in our heads can be permanently broken. And fortunately, only in the last few years have the computational abilities of the hardware and software reached a point where the tackling of this challenge was reasonably affordable.

Exactly how all this information will be used is not clear. Whether in better drug discovery through better identification of effective targets, or better knowledge of potential side-effects or predictive toxicology or metabolism, or in more subtle characterization of populations for diagnostics or prescriptions of drugs.

None the less, what is inescapable is that serious molecular and cell biology can no longer be performed without the ever-tightening integration between the life scientist and the computer.

References

1. Sonnhammer, E. L. L., Eddy, S. R., and Durbin, R. (1997). *Proteins*, **28**, 405.
2. Smith, R. F. and Smith, T. F. (1990). *Proc. Natl. Acad Sci. USA*, **87**, 118.
3. Dayhoff, M. O., Schwartz, R. M., and Orcutt, B. C. (1978). In *Atlas of protein sequence and structure* (ed. M. O. Dayhoff), pp. 345–52. National Biomedical Research Foundation, Washington, DC.
4. Sonnhammer, E. L. L. and Kahn, D. (1994). *Protein Sci.*, **3**, 482.
5. Bairoch, A. (1993). *Nucleic Acids Res.*, **21**, 3097.
6. Hunter, L., Harris, N. L., and States, D. J. (1992). *Proc. Int. Machine Learning Workshop*, pp. 224–32. Morgan Kaufman Associates, Aberdeen, Scotland.
7. Bairoch, A. (1993). *Nucleic Acids Res.*, **21**, 3155.
8. The expressed gene anatomy database (EGAD). The Institute for Genomic Research (TIGR).
9. Murzin, A. G., Brenner, S. E., Hubbard, T., and Chothia, C. (1995). *J. Mol. Biol.*, **247**, 536.
10. CATH protein classification home page. Biomolecular Structure and Modelling Unit, University College London. Dr C. A. Orengo, A. D. Michie, Dr S. Jones, Dr M. B. Swindells, Dr D. T. Jones, Prof. J. M. Thornton.
    http://www.biochem.ucl.ac.uk/bsm/cath/
11. Altschul, S. F., Gish, W., Miller, W., Myers, E. W., and Lipman, D. J. (1990). *J. Mol. Biol.*, **219**, 403.
12. Lipman, D. J. and Pearson, W. R. (1985). *Science*, **227**, 1435.
13. Smith, T. and Waterman, B. (1981). *Adv. Appl. Math.*, **2**, 482.
14. Burke, J. (1998). *Genome Res.*, **8**, 276.
15. Dawkins, R. (1989). In *The selfish gene*, p. 46. Oxford University Press.
16. Behe, M. (1996). In *Darwin's black box: the biochemical challenge to evolution*, p. 187. Touchstone Books, Simon and Schuster.
17. SNOMED (1993). *Systematized nomenclature of human and veterinary medicine.* College of American Pathology.
18. ICD 10. (1998). *International classification of diseases*, Version 10. World Health Organization.
19. CPT. (1998) *Physicians' current procedural terminology.* American Medical Association.

20. Master Drug Data Base, First DataBank, San Bruno, CA. (1998). http://www.firstdatabank.com.
21. Benson, D. A., Lipman, D. J., and Ostell, J. (1993). *Nucleic Acids Res.*, **21**, 2963.
22. Bairoch, A. and Bocckmann, B. (1991). *Nucleic Acids Res.*, **19**, 2247.
23. Tarnas, C. and Hughey, R. (1998). *Bioinformatics*, **14**, 401.
24. Karp, P. D., Riley, M., Paley, S. M., Pellegrini-Toole, A., and Krummenacker, M. (1998). *Nucleic Acids Res.*, **26**, 50.
25. Kanehisa, M. and Goto, S. (1997). In *Theoretical and computational methods in genome research* (ed. S. Suhai), pp. 41–55. Plenum Press.
26. Selkov, E., Basmanova, S., Gaasterland, T., Goryanin, I., Gretchkin, Y., Maltsev, N., *et al.* (1996). *Nucleic Acids Res.*, **24**, 26.

9

Active microelectronic arrays for DNA hybridization analysis

MICHAEL J. HELLER, EUGENE TU, ANITA HOLMSEN,
RONALD G. SOSNOWSKI, and JAMES O'CONNELL

1. Introduction

Miniaturized DNA arrays, DNA chips, and lab on a chip devices represent a new area of high technology that will revolutionize the way many important molecular biological-type experiments, assays, and tests are performed in both research and clinical diagnostic laboratories. The development of these new technologies has been brought about by a synergistic combination of diverse disciplines which include: microfabrication, organic chemistry, molecular biology, and genetics. In particular, many of these devices and technologies take advantage of sophisticated microfabrication processes developed by the semiconductor industry over the last 40 years.

Some companies are developing biochip arrays with large numbers of DNA test sites using photolithography combinatorial synthesis techniques (1–3); others are developing physical deposition methods to produce DNA arrays and improve the detection of hybrids on the DNA chip (4, 5). Still other groups are developing techniques for so-called sequencing by hybridization in microchip formats (6–8). In these devices, many parallel hybridizations occur simultaneously on immobilized oligonucleotide or other DNA probe sequences attached to the surface of the array. In most cases the hybridizations are carried out under conditions where the reaction rates and stringency conditions are controlled by temperature and salt concentration of the solutions and washes.

These more traditional 'passive' hybridization approaches have several limitations. First, since all the sequences on the array are exposed to the same conditions, the capture probes must have similar melting temperatures to achieve the same levels of hybridization stringency unless novel hybridization chemistries are employed. Secondly, as the rate of hybridization is proportional to the initial concentration of target sequence in the solution, a relatively high concentration of the target DNA is required if rapid hybridization is desired. Thirdly, the use of passive hybridization conditions for single base mismatch discrimination generally restricts one to using capture or reporter probe sequences that are generally 12–20 bases in length. Thus, passive hybridization conditions restrict or limit overall array hybridization performance in terms of speed, sensitivity, and specificity, in particular single base mismatch discriminations.

In an attempt to circumvent these limitations, Nanogen is developing microchip-based hybridization arrays that utilize electric fields as an independent parameter to:

(a) Rapidly transport and selectively address DNA probes to any position on the array surface.

(b) Accelerate the basic hybridization process.

(c) Rapidly discriminate single base mismatches in the target DNA sequences (9–12).

These DNA arrays are referred to as 'active' microelectronic devices in that they exploit both microfabrication and microelectronic technology, and that they use electric fields to directly affect the hybridization reactions. The electronic hybridization technology being developed allows many of the limitations of passive hybridization processes to be overcome, greatly improving the performance of array hybridization.

2. Background on electronic array and hybridization technology

Electronic addressing of DNA capture probes and electronic hybridization reactions are carried out by application of a DC positive bias to the individual microelectrodes beneath the selected test sites. This causes rapid electrophoretic transport and concentration of negatively charged nucleic acid molecules at the selected microlocation test sites on the microelectronic array. Nucleic acid probes (e.g. oligonucleotides, DNA, RNA, PCR amplicons, polynucleotides) are immediately immobilized (covalently or non-covalently) by direct attachment to the permeation layer overlaying the microelectrode. Similarly, the target nucleic acids can then be transported, concentrated, and hybridized to the previously addressed and attached nucleic acid probes. This rapid concentration of target DNA at the microscopic test site leads to a dramatic reduction in time for hybridization when compared to passive hybridization techniques, with the reactions occurring in seconds rather than hours.

Reversal of the electric field potential (negative bias) now causes the rapid removal of unhybridized DNA molecules. When the electric field is precisely adjusted, it affects the selective dehybridization of the DNA sequences from the attached complementary probe. This novel parameter is called 'electronic stringency' and it provides a powerful and rapid method for the discrimination of single base mismatches in target DNA sequences.

Facilitating the electronic hybridization process on the active microchip array is dependent on several other important device features and techniques. First, a crucial role is played by the permeation layer that overlies the microelectrodes. In the case of microchip-type devices, the permeation layer is a 1–2 μm coating of a hydrogel (agarose) which is spin coated over the chip surface. The permeation layer serves to protect the sensitive DNA hybridization reactions from the adverse electrochemical effects that occur on the microelectrode (platinum) surface during active operation. The permeation layer also serves as a matrix for the attachment of DNA capture probes. The structure of typical arrays and permeation layers has been described previously (10, 11). Another important consideration is the composition of the transport and hybridization buffers. To facilitate both the rapid electrophoretic transport of DNA and subsequent hybridization, buffer species that can have low conductivity states have been utilized. Histidine has been found to be particularly effective for electronic hybridization. Histidine in its zwitterionic form (near neutral pH) has low conductivity, stabilizes DNA hybridization, and maintains good buffering capacity. Histidine, in its zwitterionic state typically has a conductivity of less than 100 μS/cm, while buffers commonly employed in molecular biology have conductivities a thousand-fold greater, e.g. 6 × sodium chloride/sodium citrate.

3. Active microelectronics array fabrication

Electronically active DNA chip devices represent some of the most advanced technology in the array area. The active DNA chip device is a multisite, electronically controlled array with independently addressable test areas. Each microscopic test site is capable of attracting, binding, and repelling DNA under specific conditions of charge, polarity, current, and voltage. The chip itself is designed and constructed on silicon/silicon dioxide substrate materials using standard photolithographic techniques commonly used in the microelectronics industry. Chips with 5 × 5 arrays of 25 circular microlocations (80 μm diameter), and 10 × 10 with 100 microlocations (80 μm diameter) have been developed. Arrays with 400 or more microlocations are being developed for future applications.

Figure 1 shows a schematic representation of an electronic DNA chip with 25 addressable microlocations. The 25 microlocations are formed when the permeation layer is positioned over independently controlled platinum microelectrodes (80 μm diameter). Four auxiliary control electrodes (100 μm diameter) are positioned just outside of the main array of microelectrodes. The radiating lines are platinum wires which connect the microelectrodes to electrical contact pads on the perimeter of the device. The contact wires are covered with insulating overlayers of silicon dioxide and silicon nitride. The chip itself is about one square centimetre; the 25 active test microlocations and four auxiliary electrodes are in an area of about one square millimetre.

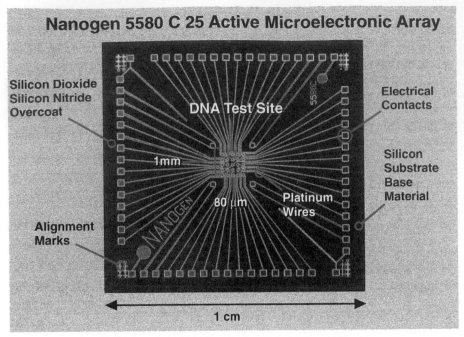

Figure 1. Schematic representation of an electronic DNA chip with 25 addressable microlocations. A permeation layer is positioned over 25 independently controlled platinum microelectrodes (80 μm diameter). Four auxiliary control electrodes (100 μm diameter) are positioned outside the main array of microelectrodes. Platinum wires connect the microelectrodes to electrical contact pads on the perimeter. Contact wires are covered with silicon dioxide and silicon nitride. Entire chips and 25 active locations are 1 cm and 1 mm, respectively.

3.1 Electronic transport, addressing, and hybridization

Electronically active DNA microarrays are able to control the transport of DNA, or for that matter any charged reagent and analyte molecules (e.g. antibodies, enzymes, cells) to or from any test site on the surface of the device. Since DNA molecules in solution carry a net negative charge, they can be moved in an electric field to any microlocation or test site area that is biased positive. This ability to transport DNA allows functionalized capture probes (e.g. biotinylated oligonucleotides, amino derivatized oligonucleotides), or other functionalized DNA/RNA sequences to be selectively attached to any microlocation test site on the chip surface. In the case of biotinylated oligonucleotide capture probes, streptavidin immobilized within the permeation layer binds the biotinylated probes to the selected test site area. Microlocations which remain unbiased (neutral), or turned to a negative bias, will not bind the capture probes.

The ability to selectively turn any one or set of test sites 'on' allows the array to be addressed with DNA probes in any desired fashion. In the DNA hybridization assay, target DNA molecules in a sample solution can now be rapidly concentrated at any positively biased microlocation test site. If the test site has a complementary DNA capture probe attached, hybridization of the target DNA can occur. The concentrating effect produced by the electric field greatly facilitates the hybridization reaction. The directed transport and addressing process can be carried out simultaneously at test sites that have different DNA capture sequences, permitting rapid multiplex analysis on a single sample. The reverse process, in which DNA is repelled from the test site by reversing the field polarity, is important to the overall hybridization specificity and sensitivity. This unique parameter is called electronic stringency control.

Electronic stringency control allows non-specific sample DNA and unhybridized probes to be selectively removed from the specific microlocation leaving the hybridized target DNA. The concept for the electronic hybridization process is illustrated in *Figure 2*. While *Figure 2* shows the so-called sandwich hybridization format, electronic hybridizations can be carried out in reverse dot blot, dot blot (with biotinylated DNA/RNA targets), and in various other formats.

3.2 Electronic stringency and base mismatch discrimination

The ability to analyse point mutations or carry out single base mismatch discrimination is critically important in many areas of genetic research and clinical diagnostics. For example, single nucleotide polymorphism (SNP) analysis will ultimately provide information regarding predisposition to diseases, as well as indicating the potential effectiveness or toxicity of drugs and therapeutics for any given individual. Many genes implicated in cancer (e.g. myc, ras, P53) are activated by point mutations, and many genetic diseases are due to single point mutations (e.g. sickle cell anaemia, thalassaemia).

Active microelectronic DNA chips have significant advantages over conventional 'passive' DNA arrays for single base mismatch analyses. By application of a negative electric field bias to a given set of test sites containing hybridized match/mismatch pairs, and adjustment of the strength of the electric field to the proper level, the match and mismatch hybrid pairs can be discriminated. This process is called 'electronic stringency' and involves an electronic dehybridization mechanism. Basically, the electric field strength is increased to the level which overcomes the binding strength of the DNA hybrid pair. Generally, this hybridization stability (binding strength) is related to the thermal melting temperature (T_m) of the hybrid pair. In most cases, the T_m increases relative to the number of bases and the percentage of G/C in the sequence.

With active DNA chips the 'electronic stringency' is precisely adjusted to correspond to the T_m of the given hybrid pair. At this point the slightly less stable mismatch sequence is dehybridized from the tethered capture probe and transported away from the test site. The loss of fluorescent signal is used

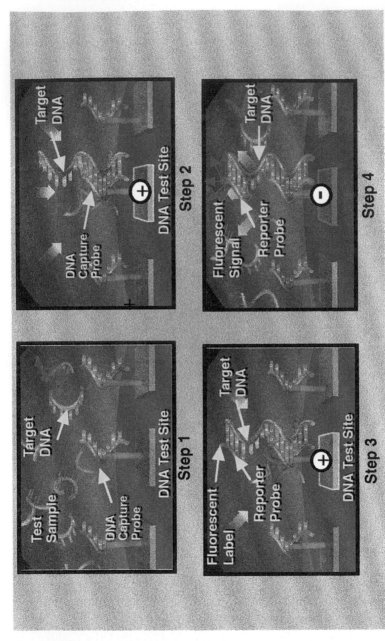

Figure 2. Concept for the electronic hybridization process. The DNA sample is applied to the chip which contains test sites for identifying specific target DNA sequences (step 1). A single DNA test sequence is shown, but an actual device contains 10^8–10^9 probe molecules. Specific test site or sites would be biased at a positive potential (step 2), causing the rapid transport, concentration, and the accelerated hybridization of the target DNA to occur at this site. Reporter probe is now attracted to the test site and hybridized to another specific portion of the target DNA molecule in a sandwich hybridization format (step 3). Following hybridization, a negative potential is applied which removes the non-specifically bound DNA from the test site (step 4).

to monitor the test sites and determine which probe/target hybrid (base pair) was mismatched. Single base mismatch discrimination analysis can be carried out in 20–30 seconds on an active DNA chip; more conventional hybridization techniques sometimes require hours to achieve similar results.

4. Point mutation analysis on active electronic arrays

The following describes the basic electronic addressing, hybridization, and stringency procedures, methods and protocols for analysis and discrimination of single base mismatches in DNA fragments. In particular, the protocols deal with the 'electronic stringency' procedures used to achieve highly selective dehybridization of mismatch sequences relative to the true match sequence. The procedures are given for carrying out base mismatch discriminations using both single-stranded fluorescent labelled DNA target sequences and fluorescent labelled PCR amplicon target sequences. Some brief descriptions are given below concerning the materials and methods for the microfabrication of the active DNA chip, permeation layer deposition, and the associated electronic control and detection instrumentation.

5. Microfabrication of active DNA chips

The following provides a brief outline of the basic process involved in the microfabrication of the 25 test site active microelectronic DNA chip. A thermal oxide (500 nm) was grown onto n-doped 4 inch silicon wafers. An optically patterned lift-off mask for electrode metalization consisted of photoresist (PR) over 1 μm of sputtered aluminium (Al). A 20 nm chrome adhesion layer was deposited and 500 nm of platinum (Pt) was deposited by e-beam process. Platinum was patterned by a lift-off process, which involves dissolving the PR in a solvent. Al was removed with an Al etch process followed by cleaning with oxygen plasma. After lift-off, a 2 μm layer of low stress silicon nitride was deposited by plasma enhanced chemical vapour deposition (PECVD). An optically patterned PR was then used as a plasma etch mask to open the microelectrode and bond pad areas. Next, the PR was removed with solvent, followed by cleaning with oxygen plasma. The chips were then coated with a third PR and diced. The last PR coating was removed with a solvent and the chips were cleaned with acetone, methanol, isopropyl, and then dried under nitrogen gas.

5.1 Permeation layer deposition

The following provides a brief description of the process used to produce the 1–2 μm permeation/attachment layer which covers the chip surface (microelectrode and surrounding test site area).

Protocol 1. Producing a permeation/attachment layer

Equipment and reagents
- 2.5% NuFix glyoxal agarose
- Streptavidin (Boehringer Mannheim)

- Spin coating apparatus EC101D (Headway Research)

Method

1. A 2.5% solution of NuFix glyoxal agarose was prepared in H_2O according to the manufacturer's protocol.

2. Streptavidin (Boehringer Mannheim) was suspended in 250 mM NaCl, 50 mM sodium phosphate pH 7.2 at 5 mg/ml and kept at room temperature (RT).

3. The boiled agarose solution was equilibrated to 65°C, then agarose and streptavidin were combined to yield 2% agarose, 1 mg/ml streptavidin.

4. 50 μl 65°C agarose was placed on a chip and spun in a spin coating apparatus at 1800 r.p.m. (18 *g*) for 20 sec, then 50 μl 65°C streptavidin/agarose is placed on this and spun at 5000 r.p.m. (140 *g*) for 20 sec at room temperature.

5. Chips were then baked at 37°C, for 30 min.

6. The Schiff's base linkage between the agarose glyoxal groups and the primary amines of streptavidin was reduced with 0.2 M sodium cyanoborohydride, 0.3 M sodium borate pH 9, at RT for 60 min.

7. Excess aldehyde groups were capped in 0.1 M glycine buffer pH 9, 30 min at RT.

8. The chips were then rinsed three times for 5 min with H_2O at RT, and then stored at 4°C.

5.2 Control and detection instrumentation

The following gives a brief description of the instrumentation that is used to control the electronic addressing and hybridization procedures, and to carry out fluorescent detection and analysis.

Protocol 2. Preparation of electronic microarray hybridization and detection station

Equipment
- Labview software (National Instruments)
- Source measure unit, 236 (Keithley)

- Relay arrays, SCXI (National Instruments)
- Epoxy ring probe card (Cerprobe)

- 594 nm HeNe lasers, ~ 10 mW (Research Electro-Optics)
- Charge-coupled detection (CCD) camera, TEC-470 (Optronics, Inc.)

Method

1. Set up a Labview virtual instrument interface to control power (current/voltage) to the electrode array from the source measure unit through an array of relays.

2. Use epoxy ring probe card mounted on a Micromanipulator Model 6000 to make connections to the chip.

3. Illuminate the chip array at an oblique angle with laser excitation by 594 nm HeNe lasers (~ 10 mW output).

4. Detect fluorescence on the test sites through an × 8 objective (0.15 numerical aperture) and 630 nm bandpass filter.

5. Collect the fluorescent hybridization signals from the test sites with a cooled, colour, charge-coupled detection (CCD) camera.

6. Acquire, quantitate, and analyse the images with NIH *Image* software on a Macintosh Power PC 8100 using a frame grabber (Data Translation or Scion).

5.3 Preparation of biotinylated and fluorescent labelled oligonucleotides

Biotinylated oligonucleotide capture probes, amino derivatized reporter probes (for subsequent fluorescent labelling), and PCR primers can be obtained from commercial sources (Oligos Etc., Inc.). If desired, these probes and primers can be synthesized using an automated DNA synthesizer, such as the ABI 380B DNA synthesizer. Oligonucleotide derivatives with 3' terminal biotin (biotin-TEG-phosphoramidite, Glen Research) can be synthesized using standard procedures supplied with the automated DNA synthesizer. Oligonucleotides with 5' terminal amino groups (C6 amino linker, Glen Research) for subsequent fluorescent labelling can be synthesized using standard procedures supplied with the automated DNA synthesizer. Bodipy Texas Red NHS ester (Molecular Probes) was used to produce the fluorescent DNA probes and primers described below. Biodipy Texas Red (ByTr) has an excitation maximum at about 594 nm and an emission maximum at about 630 nm. While the ByTr fluorophore was used in the examples below, a variety of other fluorescent labels can be used provided they can be conjugated to the oligonucleotide probe or primer sequences, and that the appropriate fluorescent detection system is available.

Michael J. Heller et al.

Protocol 3. Preparation of a Bodipy Texas Red (ByTr) conjugated oligonucleotide

Reagents
- 100–200 nmol C6 amino 5′ derivatized oligonucleotide (HPLC pure)
- 0.5 M sodium bicarbonate buffer pH 7, freshly prepared (less than one week)
- Bodipy Texas Red NHS fluorescent dye (Molecular Probes, Cat. No. D-6116)
- DMF (*N,N*-dimethylformamide) high purity spectral or HPLC grade
- Water saturated butanol mixture (upper phase is the organic)

Method

1. Concentrate the oligonucleotide to dryness in a SpeedVac (Savant Instruments). Redissolve the dried material in 40 µl deionized water (Milli-Q Water Purification System).

2. Add 12 µl 0.5 M sodium bicarbonate buffer pH 7 to the oligonucleotide solution and mix thoroughly.

3. Weigh out approx. 1.5 mg Bodipy Texas Red NHS into a microcentrifuge tube. Add 70 µl DMF and mix thoroughly.

4. Transfer the fluorescent dye/DMF to the tube containing the oligonucleotide solution and mix thoroughly. Incubate at room temperature for 2 h.

5. Removing excess dye. Add approx. 100 µl Milli-Q purified water to the tube containing the fluorescent dye/oligonucleotide reaction solution. Add 500 µl water saturated butanol (upper phase) to the reaction tube. Mix thoroughly using a vortex mixer for 20 sec. Spin the reaction tube in a microcentrifuge for 60 sec to separate the organic phase from the aqueous phase. Carefully remove the supernatant (upper organic phase) containing unreacted dye, and dispose into a waste container. Repeat until the supernatant is clear of any unreacted dye.

6. Desalt the Bodipy Texas Red (ByTr) conjugated oligonucleotide over a NAP5 column (Pharmacia) that has been equilibrated with Milli-Q purified water. Collect the dye coloured fractions.

7. The purification of the ByTr conjugated oligonucleotide is carried out using a Dynamax HPLC system (Rainin Instruments) with a C18 reverse-phase Microsorb column (Rainin; 80-220-C5).

8. The HPLC fractions containing the purified ByTr-oligonucleotide is collected and pooled, the volume is then reduced to 500 µl or less on a SpeedVac.

9. The purified ByTr-oligonucleotide is desalted over a NAP5 column that has been equilibrated with Milli-Q purified water. The fractions containing the coloured product are collected.

10. The concentration of the purified ByTr-oligonucleotide is determined by measuring the absorbance at 260 nm, 280 nm, and 594 nm on a UV-VIS spectrophotometer. Final quality control or purity analysis can be verified by either analytical HPLC or polyacrylamide gel electrophoresis.

5.4 Addressing capture oligonucleotides to the microchip array

Addressing of biotinylated capture oligonucleotide probes or other biotinylated DNA or RNA sequences to the microchip array is carried out by contacting the array with the biotinylated capture probe sequence in a zwitterionic histidine buffer (50 mM, pH 7.4) solution. Generally, the concentration of the capture probe can be from 50–500 nM for the addressing procedure. In some cases, several test sites on the array are pre-addressed with a fluorescent control probe. This probe is a homologous 12-mer sequence of thymidine derivatized in the 3' terminal position with a biotin and in the 5' terminal position with the Bodipy Texas Red (ByTr) fluorescent dye. The biotin-T12-ByTr control probe servers as an indicator that the electronic addressing procedure is functioning, and is occurring specifically at the test site(s) being addressed.

For single base mismatch discrimination analysis in the reverse dot blot format, capture probes sequences from 20–26 bases in length are generally used (this does not exclude using probes less than 20 bases in length). Depending on the application (point mutations or SNPs) from two to four biotinylated capture probes are used to discriminate the mismatched base in the target sequence. The two probe discrimination system would include a matched base probe and a second probe containing the most common mismatched base for that point mutation, while in the four probe discrimination system each probe would have one of the four bases (A, T, G, and C). The matched and mismatched discrimination base is usually placed at or near the middle of the probe sequence.

Protocol 4. Electronic microarray hybridization and detection

Equipment and reagents
- STAR instrument system
- Zwitterionic histidine buffer (50 mM, pH 7.4)
- Biotinylated T12 ByTr fluorescent control probe, 50 nM

Method

1. The 25 test site active microchip array is positioned on either the electronic controller workstation or the STAR instrument system.

2. The array is washed three times with 20 µl aliquots of zwitterionic histidine buffer (50 mM, pH 7.4).

Protocol 4. *Continued*

3. The array is now contacted with 20 μl 50 nM biotinylated T12 ByTr fluorescent control probe in a zwitterionic histidine buffer (50 mM, pH 7.4). Generally, the fluorescent control probe is addressed to the 1,1 and 5,5 test sites on the 25 test site chip (considering the test sites to be in a five column and five row arrangement, with upper left hand being the 1,1 site).

4. The two test sites are biased positive at 200 nA/pad (400 nA total current) for 1 min, relative to the negatively biased four corner control electrodes.

5. The array is now washed five times with 20 μl aliquots of zwitterionic histidine buffer (50 mM, pH 7.4).

6. Under fluorescent observation (594 nm excitation and 630 nm emission) the 1,1 and 5,5 test sites should produce a high fluorescent signal, while the unaddressed test sites remain dark (no fluorescent signal).

7. Biotinylated capture probes can now be addressed in either serial (one specific probe sequence per test site) or in a parallel fashion (one specific probe sequence to multiple test sites). The array is contacted with 20 μl of 500 nM solution of the first biotinylated oligonucleotide capture probe in zwitterionic histidine buffer (50 mM, pH 7.4). The first capture probe is addressed to the desired test site by positively biasing the site at 200 nA/pad for 1 min, relative to the negatively biased four corner control electrodes. If multiple test sites are being addressed, the current level (nA) is increased proportionally. For example, if three test sites are being addressed, a total of 600 nA would be used for 1 min. The array is now washed five times with zwitterionic histidine buffer (50 mM, pH 7.4).

8. The process is repeated until all the desired capture probe sequences have been addressed to their selected test sites. The array is washed a final five times with zwitterionic histidine buffer (50 mM, pH 7.4), and is now ready for hybridization.

5.5 Electronic hybridization and stringency

Hybridization of target DNA sequences to the active microchip array can be carried out using either active electronic or passive procedures. Generally, if the target concentration in the sample is low ($< 10^8$ copies), then an active electronic procedure would be used to accelerate the hybridization rate and reduce the overall assay time. The active electronic hybridization procedure is also useful in cases where there is a relatively high concentration of double-stranded target material, but the sample has a low DNA complexity background (fully amplified PCR reactions). In this case, the competition from the presence of the complementary DNA strands greatly reduces the efficiency of the hybridization of the target strands to the capture probes on the array. DNA arrays that are restricted to passive hybridization procedures often require isolation of single-stranded target before base mismatch analysis can be carried out.

Electronic hybridization in low conductance zwitterionic histidine buffer overcomes this problem; and PCR amplicons can be directly hybridized to the array without the need to isolate single-stranded material. A fluorescent label can be incorporated into the PCR amplicon target strand by using a ByTr labelled PCR primer for the PCR reaction. In those cases where there is a high concentration of single-stranded target material ($> 10^9$ copies), the more conventional passive hybridization procedures can be used to carry out the assays in a reasonable time period. Single-stranded target DNA sequences can either be labelled directly with the ByTr fluorescent dye or hybridized with a secondary reporter probe which is fluorescently labelled.

After hybridization of the target DNA to the array, the process called 'electronic stringency' is used to affect the rapid discrimination of single base mismatches on the array. In this process a precisely controlled negative electric field produced at the test sites is used to cause the selective dehybridization of the target DNA strand from the mismatched capture probe site relative to the matched capture probe site. The electric field strength is increased to a level that just overcomes the binding strength of the mismatch DNA hybrid pair, causing it to dehybridize and transport away from the test site.

Electronic stringency is measured in terms of the current level or nanoamperes (nA) that are delivered to the negatively biased test site over a given period of time (20–40 sec). Generally, the electronic stringency or current level (nA) used to affect the dehybridization of a given hybrid pair is proportional to its thermal melting temperature (T_m). Thus, a hybrid pair with a T_m of 45 °C might have an electronic stringency level of 500 nA, while a hybrid pair with a T_m of 70 °C might have an electronic stringency level of 900 nA. While the absolute current levels for a given electronic stringency can vary due to other variables and chip characteristics, the relative differences remain constant. The active electronic hybridization and electronic stringency procedure for fully amplified PCR targets is given in *Protocol 5*. The passive hybridization and electronic stringency procedure for single-stranded targets is given in *Protocol 6*.

Protocol 5. Electronic hybridization/stringency for PCR targets

Reagents
- Zwitterionic histidine buffer (50 mM, pH 7.4)

Method
1. 1–2 µl from an amplified PCR reaction is diluted into 100 µl zwitterionic histidine buffer (50 mM, pH 7.4).

Protocol 5. *Continued*

2. The capture probe addressed array is pre-washed three times with 20 μl aliquots of zwitterionic histidine buffer (50 mM, pH 7.4).

3. The array is contacted with 20 μl of the diluted PCR reaction.

4. The desired hybridization test sites are biased positive at 600 nA/ site for 2 min, relative to the negatively biased four corner control electrodes.

5. The array is now washed five times with 20 μl aliquots of zwitterionic histidine buffer (50 mM, pH 7.4).

6. The electronic hybridization procedure can be repeated for other PCR targets or samples which can be selectively hybridized to other test sites on the array.

7. The array is washed three times with 20 μl aliquots of zwitterionic histidine buffer (50 mM, pH 7.4). A pre-stringency fluorescent image is taken of the array.

8. The array is washed ten times with 20 μl aliquots of 20 mM sodium phosphate, 20 mM Tris buffer at pH 9.5 (stringency buffer). The last aliquot is left on the array.

9. Electronic stringency is now carried out by negatively biasing the desired match/mismatched test sites relative to the positively biased control electrodes, and pulsing the appropriate electronic stringency current (400 nA/site to 1.2 μA/site) for 150 cycles at 0.1 sec on/ 0.1 sec off.

10. The array is washed three times with 20 μl aliquots of 20 mM sodium phosphate, 20 mM Tris buffer at pH 9.5.

11. Fluorescent detection (594 nm excitation and 630 nm emission) and imaging analysis of the chip is now carried out.

Protocol 6. Passive hybridization/electronic stringency for single-stranded target

1. The capture probe addressed array is pre-washed with a 20 μl aliquot of 40 mM sodium phosphate, 500 mM NaCl buffer at pH 7.5.

2. Samples of between 5–20 μl, containing single-stranded target DNA sequences in concentration ranges from 10 nM to 10 μM are made up in 40 mM sodium phosphate, 500 mM NaCl buffer at pH 7.5.

3. A 5–20 μl sample containing the single-stranded target DNA sequence is placed on the array and hybridized at RT for 2–20 min (depending on target concentration).

4. The array is washed ten times with 20 μl aliquots of 40 mM sodium phosphate, 500 mM NaCl buffer at pH 7.5.

5. The array is washed ten times with 20 μl aliquots of 20 mM sodium phosphate, 20 mM Tris buffer at pH 9.5 (stringency buffer). The last aliquot is left on the array and a pre-stringency fluorescent image is taken.

6. Electronic stringency is now carried out by negatively biasing the desired match/mismatched test sites relative to the positively biased control electrodes, and pulsing the appropriate electronic stringency current (400 nA/site to 1.2 μA/site) for 150 cycles at 0.1 sec on/ 0.1 sec off.

7. The array is washed three times with 20 μl aliquots of 20 mM sodium phosphate, 20 mM Tris buffer at pH 9.5.

8. Fluorescent imaging analysis (594 nm excitation and 630 nm emission) of the chip is now carried out.

6. Example of single base discrimination analysis

The following describes single base mismatch experimental results that were achieved using the active 25 test site microelectronic chip to carry out electronic addressing, hybridization, and stringency for P53 exon 8 single-stranded target sequences. Generally, these single-stranded target sequences are used to determine the electronic stringency level that is necessary for the given match/mismatch hybrid pairs. In this example, four capture probes were used that were biotinylated 24-mer sequences, specific for a single base mismatch in exon 8 of the P53 tumour suppressor gene. The DNA target was a 5′ labelled fluorescent Bodipy Texas Red 51-mer sequence, in which the match base was a C residue. The target DNA sequence was completely complementary (an exact match) to the No. 4 G capture probe; a one base mismatch with capture probes No. 1 (C), No. 2 (A), and No. 3 (T); and completely non-complementary to the ATA5 capture probe, which served as a negative control. The base sequence of all the capture probes and the target are shown in *Table 1*.

Passive hybridization and electronic stringency were carried out according to *Protocol 6*. For the P53 exon 8 hybrid pairs in rows 1 through 4, the optimal electronic stringency level of 700 nA/site was applied for 30 sec. For the P53 exon 8 hybrid pairs in row 5, a higher than optimal electronic stringency level of 800 nA/site was applied for 30 sec. The results for these experiments are shown in *Figure 3*. *Figure 3* shows the actual fluorescent images of the array both before and after electronic stringency was applied. *Figure 4* shows image analysis of the fluorescent signal intensity at each test site, presented as three-dimensional colour intensity peaks. Before electronic stringency is applied

181

Table 1. P53 exon 8 capture probes and target sequence[a]

No.	Type	Sequence
1	Capture	5′-CAG-GCA-CAA-ACA-[C]GC-ACC-TCA-AAG-3′-Biotin
2	Capture	5′-CAG-GCA-CAA-ACA-[A]GC-ACC-TCA-AAG-3′-Biotin
3	Capture	5′-CAG-GCA-CAA-ACA-[T]GC-ACC-TCA-AAG-3′-Biotin
4	Capture	5′-CAG-GCA-CAA-ACA-[G]GC-ACC-TCA-AAG-3′-Biotin
1	Target	ByTr-5′-AA-CAG-CTT-TGA-GGT-GC[C]-TGT-TTG-TGC-CTG-TCC-TGG-GGA-GAG-ACC-GGC-GCA-CA-3′
1	Control	5′-G-ATG-AGC-AGT-TCT-ACG-TGG-Biotin

[a] The capture probes were addressed to the array according to the procedure in *Protocol 4*; with capture probe No. 1 **[C]** being addressed to the five test sites in column 1; capture probe No. 2 **[A]** being addressed to the five test sites in column 2; capture probe No. 3 **[T]** being addressed to the five test sites in column 3; capture probe No. 4 **[G]** being addressed to the five test sites in column 4; and the ATA5 non-complementary control probe being addressed to the five test sites in column 5.

both the match and mismatch test sites in columns 1 through 4 show the same relative levels of fluorescent signal intensity (hybridization).

However, the non-complementary ATA5 probe in the column 5 test sites shows very little hybridization signal. After optimal electronic stringency was applied to rows 1 through 4, the fluorescent signal intensity was observed to decrease for the mismatched hybrids (C-C, C-A, C-T) in columns 1 through 3, but remained significantly higher for the matched hybrid pair (G-C) in column 4.

P53 Exon 8 Point Mutations Before and After Electronic Stringency (Fluorescent Array Image)

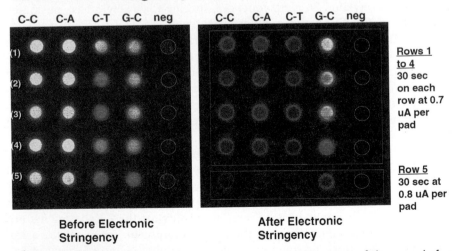

Figure 3. P53 exon 8 point mutation detection. Fluorescent images of the array before (left panel) and after electronic stringency (right panel) are shown. Electronic stringency level of 700 nA/site was applied for 30 sec (row 1–4) or 800 nA/site for 30 sec (row5).

P53 Exon 8 Point Mutations Before and After Electronic Stringency (Color Image Intensity Analysis)

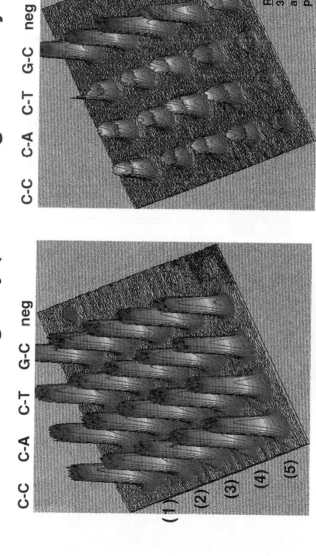

Before Electronic Stringency

After Electronic Stringency

Figure 4. Image intensity analysis of point mutation detection. Image analysis of the fluorescent signal intensity at each test site, presented as three-dimensional colour intensity peaks. Control probe (column 5) shows very low hybridization signal. Before and after electronic stringency is shown in the left and right panels, respectively.

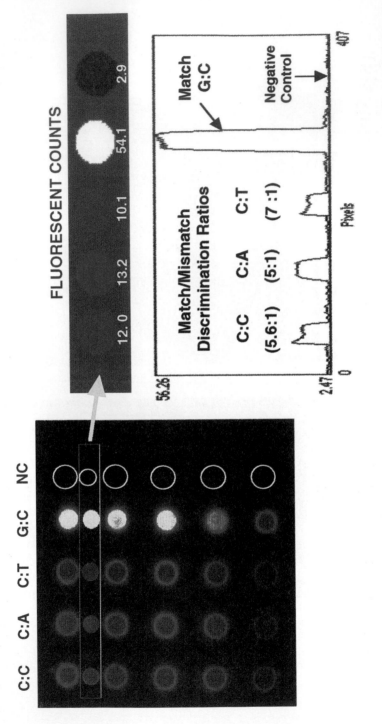

Figure 5. Quantitative data analysis of point mutation analysis. Discrimination ratios for each of the match/mismatch ratios was determined (C-C = 5.6 to 1, C-A = 5 to 1, and C-T = 7 to 1).

The fluorescent signal intensities in row 5 (including the G-C matched hybrid), are all greatly reduced after the higher than optimal electronic stringency was applied. *Figure 5* shows the results of further quantitative data analysis, where the discrimination ratios for each of the match/mismatch ratios was determined (C-C = 5.6 to 1, C-A = 5 to 1, and C-T = 7 to 1).

7. Conclusions

Active electronic microchip array technology offers a number of distinct advantages for DNA hybridization analysis and differentiates itself from other 'passive chip' technologies by providing:

(a) Electronic addressing which allows selective transport of DNA molecules by charge.

(b) Electronic hybridization for concentration effect which improves the DNA hybridization rate.

(c) Electronic stringency control, which improves selectivity and allows rapid discrimination of single base pair mismatches.

References

1. Fodor, S. P. A., Read, J. L., Pirrung, M. C., Stryer, L., Lu, A. T., and Solas, D. (1991). *Science*, **251**, 767.
2. Fodor, S. P., Rava, R. P., Huang, X. C., Pease, A. C., Holmes, C. P., and Adams, C. L. (1993). *Nature*, **364**, 555.
3. Chee, M., Yang, R., Hubbell, E., Berno, A., Huang, X. C., Stern, D., *et al.* (1996). *Science*, **274**, 610.
4. Eggers, M., Hogan, M., Reich, R. K., Lamture, J., Ehrlich, D., Hollis, M., *et al.* (1994). *Biotechniques*, **17**, 516.
5. Lamture, J. B., Beattie, K. L., Burke, B. E., Eggers, M. D., Ehrlich, D. J., Fowler, R., *et al.* (1994). *Nucleic Acids Res.*, **22**, 2121.
6. Bains, W. and Smith, G. C. (1988). *J. Theor. Biol.*, **135**, 303.
7. Drmanac, R., Labat, L., Brukner, I., and Crkvenjakov, R. (1989). *Genomics*, **4**, 114.
8. Southern, E. M., Maskos, U., and Elder, J. K. (1992). *Genomics*, **13**, 1008.
9. Heller, M. J. (1996). *IEEE Eng. Med. Biol.*, **15**, 100.
10. Sosnowski, R. G., Tu, E., Butler, W. F., O'Connell, J. P., and Heller, M. J. (1997). *Proc. Natl. Acad. Sci. USA*, **94**, 1119.
11. Edman, C. F., Raymond, D. E., Wu, D. J., Tu, E., Sosnowski, R. G., Butler, W. F., *et al.* (1997). *Nucleic Acids Res.*, **25**, 4907.
12. Cheng, J., Sheldon, E. L., Wu, L., Uribe, A., Gerrue, L. O., Carrino, J., *et al.* (1998). *Nature Biotechnol.*, **16**, 541.

10

Gene chips and microarrays: applications in disease profiles, drug target discovery, drug action and toxicity

RENU A. HELLER, JOHN ALLARD, FENGRONG ZUO,
CHRISTOPHER LOCK, STACY WILSON, PAUL KLONOWSKI,
HANS GMUENDER, HAROLD VAN WART, and ROBERT BOOTH

1. Introduction

The high density microchips and microarrays are novel technologies. They provide the ability to query the action patterns of hundreds and thousands of genes simultaneously (1–6) and therefore allow parallel genetic analyses. Not only can they furnish gene expression profiles during normal development and differentiation, they can also provide a view of the disease state and its progression. Complex diseases, in particular, are difficult to comprehend because of the multiplicity of factors involved such as different cell types, cell type-specific gene expression, altered expression patterns caused by a malfunctioning of autocrine or paracrine controls, and so on. With parallel genetic analysis, normal gene expression patterns and those gone awry can be traced to provide a level of comprehension heretofore not feasible.

Recently several novel methods have been developed to assess gene expression patterns (1–3, 6–8). In the development of therapeutic drugs, these technologies lend themselves to many applications including drug target discovery, human disease profiles, evaluation of animal models of human disease, tests for drug efficacy, specificity, and toxicity. Readouts of parallel genetic information are indicative of the functions altered, the specific signalling pathways affected, and responses altered as a consequence of drug action. The two commercial technologies most widely used are the Synteni microarrays and the Affymetrix gene chips. The questions frequently raised are the relative ease of applying these technologies, their sensitivity, reproducibility, and speed. We have used both of these technologies to look at gene expression profiles of cell lines and diseased tissue and consider them largely as complementary technologies as detailed below.

However, gene expression technologies are a challenge to use. They are not of 'plug and play' simplicity and are also very expensive. Access to and application of the technologies provides tools to interrogate physiological processes that result in overwhelming amounts of data, not necessarily information. Evaluation of the disease state requires a comprehension of these massive amounts of data to provide the understanding, insights, and perspectives. This indeed is a challenge for the post-genomics era. Nevertheless, the advantages of the microarrays and gene chips are the speed of investigation, economy of reagents, and the ability to observe gene action in unison. In this article, in addition to the frequently raised questions of chip design, sample preparation, sensitivity of the technologies, and reproducibility of data, their many applications will also be commented upon.

2. Methods

2.1 Synteni microarray and sample preparation

Detailed information on the Synteni microarrays can be best obtained from the company (10). For preparation of the microarrays sequences from the 3′ end of the genes are preferable for spotting or attaching to the chip. These target DNAs are prepared from individual clones of cDNA by PCR amplification and spotted onto derivatized glass slides (2, 4). Currently, the minimum target length and concentration of these PCR products required for spotting is 500 bp as a 1 µg/µl solution. At this concentration target abundance for hybridization to even highly expressed messages does not become limiting. For preparing the Synteni microarrays from an expression library cDNA inserts can be amplified by PCR and arrayed without knowledge of sequence, identity, or function. Duplication of clones on the array can be avoided by prior single pass sequencing when expressed sequence tags or ESTs can be identified by BLAST analysis against sequence databases. Single pass sequencing of approximately 10 000 colonies from a library is generally enough to select 1000–2000 unique clones for arraying. Also, by initially obtaining clones from a subtraction library of diseased and untreated or normal tissue, the enrichment for differentially expressed genes can be enhanced. Therefore, microarrays representing any chosen biological state can be made. It is also possible to select known cDNA or genomic clones representing one or more classes of genes, amplify unique gene-specific target sequences, and use them to prepare microarrays defining one or more functional class of molecules, for example the kinases, phosphatases, cell surface receptors, etc.

The hybridizing sample contains antisense cDNA transcribed from mRNA isolated from biological samples with an oligo(dT) primer. The processivity of reverse transcriptase is critical for the length of cDNA transcribed and it can be adversely affected by the incorporation of modified nucleotides required to label the sample. These modified nucleotides are fluoro-linked dCTP molecules.

In their presence, the average length of the cDNA transcribed is around 1.5 kb which means that upon hybridization signals are primarily generated by the 3' end half of the genes. It is well known that a hallmark of this technique is the simultaneous hybridization of two cDNA samples containing different fluorescent nucleotides to the same microarray to allow suitable comparisons.

2.2 Affymetrix chip design and sample preparation

For Affymetrix gene expression chip design, as with Synteni microarrays, the preferable region to represent the gene with is again the 3' rather than the 5' half. Information on the technology can be best obtained from the company itself (11). It is well known that the Affymetrix chips have 25-mer oligonucleotide sequences of the gene tiled as probes directly on the solid glass wafer. The probes are organized as perfect match/mismatch pairs, with the mismatch probe acting as a control for hybridization specificity. Unique regions for individual genes can be specified for a class of genes. Currently as little as 20 probe pairs per gene can be used for expression analysis, which for 25 nucleotides per probe pair requires a minimum of 500 nucleotides of unique sequence per gene or its related family member. With 20 probe pairs per gene, the density of genes per chip has increased to 1600. Further reduction in feature size (the area occupied by each collection of 25-mers) allows the density of the chip to reach over 6000 genes per chip. Clearly, a major difference between preparation of the Synteni microarrays and Affymetrix gene chips is the absolute necessity of the nucleotide sequence for the *in situ* synthesis of genes on the Affymetrix chips. Only sequence information is required, and the handling of clones, PCR products, etc. is not involved. The probes are short oligonucleotides and can be designed to discriminate splice variants, members of gene families, etc. Samples for hybridization to Affymetrix chips are antisense copy RNA (cRNA) made *in vitro* in the presence of biotinylated ribonucleotides Bio-CTP and Bio-UTP. The antisense cRNA is made from double-stranded cDNA derived from tissue mRNA. After hybridization of the biotinylated cRNA, the chip is stained with streptavidin–phycoerythrin and read with a scanning confocal microscope.

2.3 Preparation of RNA from cell lines and tissues

RNA is used for sample preparation for both technologies. The procedures for RNA preparation from cell lines and tissues are well established (11). Problems are encountered frequently with fresh tissue as the source or with tissue frozen in liquid nitrogen. Depending upon the type of tissue, difficulties can be due to impermeability of the tissue to RNA extraction reagents, e.g. phenol, guanidinium isothiocyanate, or guanidinium hydrochloride. Delayed action results in degradation of the RNA, lowered yields, and erroneous results. For post-mortem human tissue, material obtained from an early autopsy performed within 2–4 h is dramatically different from one done at a later time.

The latter shows drastically reduced expression levels that are most likely due to tissue degradation and loss of RNA. For best results samples obtained at surgery should be frozen in liquid nitrogen as they are dissected. For tissue samples the following protocol works well.

Protocol 1. RNA isolation from tissue with TRIZOL reagent

This protocol is adapted from the Gibco BRL instructions for RNA isolation.

Equipment and reagents

- TRIZOL
- Conical screw-cap polypropylene tube (VWR, Cat. No. 21008-178)
- Tissue homogenizer, pt 10/35 (Brinkmann)

- Oakridge polypropylene tube (Labcor Inc., Cat. No. 112-143)
- Phase Lock Gel III, heavy (5'→3' Inc., Cat. No. p1-982148)

Method

1. Immediately after dissection, freeze the tissue quickly by placing it into liquid nitrogen. Cut large size tissue (e.g. brain, lung) into smaller pieces before freezing.

2. For RNA extraction, use a ratio of 10 ml TRIZOL per gram of tissue.

3. Grind the tissue with a tissue homogenizer (Brinkmann) in a conical tube (VWR or Labcor) kept in ice. For softer tissues, several 15 sec pulses are enough, but for more intransigent tissues like tendon or artery, several 30 sec pulses work better. When working with multiple samples, wash the probe between samples with a 1:1 mixture of 100% ethanol and fresh TRIZOL reagent.

4. Shake the blended sample vigorously and centrifuge for 10 min at 10 000 g.

5. Transfer the supernatant to a fresh Oakridge or VWR tube. Incubate the sample at room temperature for 5 min.

6. Add 0.2 ml chloroform/1 ml TRIZOL reagent.

7. Seal the tube securely and shake sample vigorously for 15 sec.

8. Incubate at room temperature for 2–3 min.

9. Centrifuge at 12 000 g for 15 min at 4°C in a JA-20 rotor with GSA adapters for conical-bottom Oakridge tubes. The mixture should separate into a lower red phenol:chloroform phase, an interphase, and a colourless upper aqueous phase. The top aqueous layer should be approximately 60% of the original volume of TRIZOL reagent used for homogenization.

10. Remove the top aqueous layer to an RNase-free centrifuge tube. Alternatively, 50 ml conical tubes containing Phase Lock Gel III

($5'{\rightarrow}3'$) can be used, in which case the chloroform:TRIZOL mixture is transferred to the Phase Lock tube, kept at room temperature for 5 min, and the tube centrifuged at 4000 g for 5–15 min in a swinging-bucket rotor to separate the organic phase (under the Phase Lock interface) from the RNA-containing upper phase.

11. Total RNA is precipitated by adding 0.5 ml isopropanol/1 ml TRIZOL used in the original homogenization step.

12. Contents are mixed and incubated at room temperature for 5 min.

13. Pellet the RNA by centrifugation at 12000 g for 10 min at 4°C. The supernatant is carefully decanted and discarded.

14. Rinse the RNA pellet with 75% ethanol (made with DEPC treated water).

15. Resuspend the RNA pellet in 400 μl DEPC treated water.

16. Transfer the RNA sample to an RNase-free microcentrifuge tube.

17. Mix with an equal volume of 25:24:1 phenol:chloroform:isoamyl alcohol (saturated with 10 mM Tris–HCl pH 8/1 mM EDTA) (Gibco). The entire total RNA–phenol:chloroform mixture is added to a Phase Lock Gel tube centrifuged prior to sample addition in a micro-centrifuge for 20–30 sec (1.5 ml tube with PLG I-light, $5'{\rightarrow}3'$ Inc.) and centrifuged at full speed (12000 g or higher) for 2 min. The upper aqueous phase is transferred to fresh RNase-free 1.5 ml tube and the RNA precipitated by adding 0.1 vol. 3 M sodium acetate (RNase-free; Sigma) and 0.8 vol. isopropanol (RNA vol. plus sodium acetate vol.), mixed by inversion, and stored at –20°C for at least 0.5 h. The sample is centrifuged at full speed in a microcentrifuge for 20 min, the pellet rinsed with 75% ethanol, respun at full speed in a microcentrifuge for 5 min, and resuspended in 0.2–0.4 ml DEPC treated water. Quantitation of RNA can be done with a Beckman DU series spectrophotometer (e.g. DU-70) which uses microcells in a Micro Auto-1 Accessory. These microcells take only 50 μl of solution and are ideal for small (0.5–1 μl) aliquots of RNA solutions for quantitation. Total RNA can be dissolved in 20–400 μl water depending upon the expected amount and aiming for a 1–2 μg/μl concentration. The amount of RNA is quantitated by its dual wavelength absorbance at 260 nm and 280 nm (12). Purification of 2 × mRNA from total RNA was done with the Qiagen Oligotex kit. cDNA and *in vitro* transcribed RNA were prepared with Gibco BRL and Ambion reagents, and procedures provided by Synteni or Affymetrix.

2.4 Bioinformatics and data analysis

This is a component of the parallel genetic analysis that has lagged behind the experimental laboratory work. It is being rapidly developed and is critical because reams of data are produced by the microarray and gene chip technologies that can become totally unmanageable. In-house expertise is required to evaluate, develop, and adopt programs, and set up relational databases to develop and utilize software acquired. Synteni's GemTools and Affymetrixís LIMS are tools being developed for this purpose.

3. Results

Over the past few years several publications have introduced the use of the Synteni and Affymetrix technologies (1, 2, 5, 6, 9). Here we provide some comparative data on the two technologies, and the frequently asked questions on their applications and preferential use.

The genes on the Synteni microarray are shown in *Figure 1* and are similar to an earlier 96 gene array (7) on which several inflammatory disease tissues were screened. To compare the two technologies, this panel of genes was also synthesized as a component of an Affymetrix chip using 60 oligonucleotide probe pairs for each gene, as shown in *Figure 2*. Basically, the two sets of arrays with identical genes, *Figures 1* and *2*, provided us with platforms for comparison of the Synteni and Affymetrix technologies.

	1	2	3	4	5	6	7	8	9	10	11	12
A	HAT1 control1	HAT4 control2	HAT4 control2	MBP MBP	HPRT HPRT	UBQ Ubiquitin	IL12A IL-12A	BMP1 BMP-1	BMPHIS BMP-1/HIS	BMPTLD BMP-1/Tld	BMPHIS BMP-1/HIS	
B	IL1A IL-1a	IL1B IL-1b	IL1RA IL-1RA	IL2 IL-2	IL3 IL-3	IL4 IL-4	IL6 IL-6	IL6R IL-6R	IL7 IL-7	CFOS c-fos	CJUN c-jun	CREL c-rel
C	IL8 IL-8	IL9 IL-9	IL10 IL-10	ICE ICE	IFNG IFN-g	GCSF G-CSF	MCSF M-CSF	GMCSF GM-CSF	TNFB.1 TNFb	CREB2 CREB2	NFKB50 NFkBp50	NFKB65.1 NFkBp65
D	TNFA.1 TNFa	TNFA.2 TNFa	TNFA.3 TNFa	TNFA.4 TNFa	TNFA.5 TNFa	TNFRI.1 TNFrI	TNFRI.2 TNFrI	TNFRII.1 TNFrII	TNFRII.2 TNFrII	NFKB65.2 NFkBp65	IKB IkB	RFRA1 rFra-1
E	STR1 Str-1	STR2-3' Str-2	STR3 Str-3	COL1 Col-1	COL1-3' Col-1	COL2.1 Col-2	COL2.2 Col-2	COL3 Col-3	COX1 Cox-1	COX2 Cox-2	12LO 12-LO	15LO 15-LO
F	GELA.1 GelA	GELB GelB	HNE Elastase	MTMMP MT-MMP	PUMP1 Matrilysin	TIMP1 TIMP-1	TIMP2 TIMP-2	TIMP3 TIMP-3	ICAM1 ICAM	VCAM VCAM	LDLR LDLR	INOS INOS
G	EGF EGF	FGFA FGF acidic	FGFB FGF basic	IGFI IGF-I	IGFII IGF-II	TGFA TGFa	TGFB TGFb	PDGFB PDGFb	CALCTN Calcitonin	GH1 GH-1	GRO GRO	GCR Gluc.Rec
H	MCP1.1 MCP-1	MCP1.2 MCP-1	MIP1A MIP-1a	MIP1B MIP-1b	MIF MIF	RANTES RANTES	BACTIN b-actin	G3PDH G3PDH	ALU.1 IL-10	ALU.2 TNFrII	ALU.3 IL-10 cds+alu	POLYA poly-A

Figure 1. The 96-element microarray design. The target element name and the corresponding gene are shown in the layout. Some genes have more than one target sequence in order to guarantee specificity of signal. For TNF the targets represent decreasing lengths of 1 kb, 0.8 kb, 0.6 kb, 0.4 kb, and 0.2 kb, from left to right.

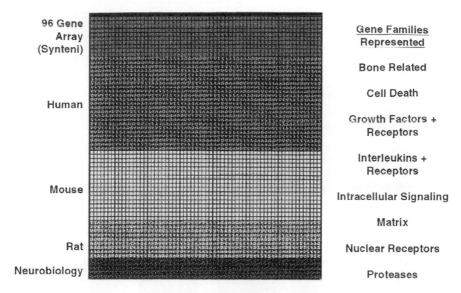

Figure 2. A diagrammatic representation of the genes on an Affymetrix-500 gene chip. This chip has a block of genes that are the same as the Synteni 96-gene microarray. On this Affymetrix chip, there are 295 human genes, 127 mouse genes, and 80 rat genes. They fall into various functional classes related to bone metabolism, cell death, growth factors and receptors, interleukins and receptors, intracellular signalling, matrix, nuclear receptors, and proteases.

However, given the access to these technologies, in order to take full advantage of them, in-house facilities and expertise are also required. These include a bioinformatics infrastructure for selection of desired genes or DNA sequences from databases, and a source for obtaining genes for Synteni microarrays, and nucleotide sequences of the genes to be built on the Affymetrix chips. EST sequence databases are rapidly increasing in volume and the ability to assemble, align, select, and array novel open reading frames is a valuable routine to acquire and obtain novel genes. Open reading frame sequences can be obtained from cDNA or genomic libraries, or even derived by PCR from known sources. Proficiency to develop dependable analytical tools linked to data visualization programs, plus the skills to retrieve and display data is another useful talent. Bioinformatics know how, software tools, and databases were developed in-house or acquired for the applications of these technologies (*Figure 3*). These tools can be obtained from the biotechnology companies as well, but a reasonable time and effort is needed up front for both the hardware and software set ups, provided the expertise to operate them is at hand.

An earlier study with the Synteni microarrays had examined cell lines, a human monocytic cell Mono Mac 6 and a chondrosarcoma cell line SW1352. These were treated with inducing agents, either lipopolysaccharide and phorbol

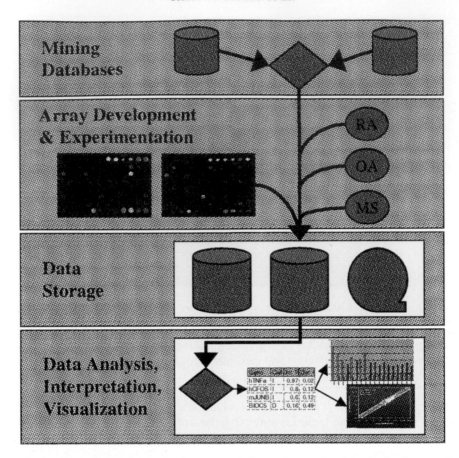

Figure 3. Databases for storage of sequence information, retrieval, and selection require software programs for sequence organization, for PCR primer selection, documentation of amplification products, arraying patterns, display and analysis of data. Large capacity servers linked to workstations for information storage and analysis are part of the essential hardware that utilizes software programs still very much in the development stages to mine the reams of data obtained with these technologies. Here OA, RA, and MS refer to tissue from osteoarthritis, rheumatoid arthritis, and multiple sclerosis, and represent the disease under investigation.

myristate acetate, or tumour necrosis factor and interleukin-β respectively (7). We repeated this study, and prepared total RNA and poly(A) RNA. Half the yield was saved for gene expression analysis with the Synteni microarrays as described earlier, while the other half was purified one more time to give 2 × purified mRNA. This was further processed according to protocols provided by Affymetrix to make cDNA and transcribed *in vitro* to make copy RNA. Biotinylated UTP and CTP ribonucleotides were incorporated during this reaction using T7 RNA polymerase and the purified samples were

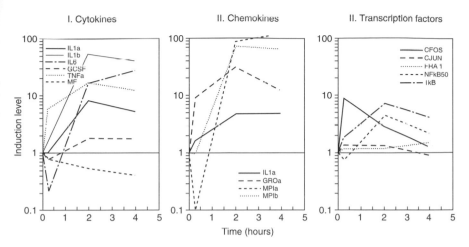

Figure 4. Time course for LPS and PMA-induced Mono Mac 6 cells. The gene activities profiled above were determined with Affymetrix gene chips on which each gene was synthesized as 60 probe pairs, each 25 nucleotides long in a 50 μm × 50 μm feature, each containing ~ 10⁷ molecules. Total RNA was isolated from the cells at the indicated times after induction and was used to prepare the hybridizing samples containing biotinylated copy RNA made *in vitro*, according to protocols provided by Affymetrix. Chips were hybridized, stained with streptavidin–phycoerythrin, and scanned for fluorescence intensity using a scanning confocal microscope. Data processing used Affymetrix gene chip software and functional hierarchy developed at Roche for mining classes of genes, and displayed using software programs developed in-house.

hybridized to the chips, stained with streptavidin–phycoerythrin, and scanned for fluorescence intensity with a scanning confocal microscope. Results from both microarray and gene chip technologies were compared with values obtained with the traditional methods of dot blot and Northern blot analysis. The results from the Synteni arrays were not different from those reported earlier (7), so that we have omitted them from this report and included only the data from the gene chip experiments and blotting methods (*Figures 4* and *5* and *Table 1*). The earlier publication can be consulted for data with Synteni microarrays (7).

Using the same sample and the different techniques mentioned above, the activities of several different genes were measured. In general the pattern of change obtained with the two techniques was consistent (*Figures 4* and *5*) both for the Mono Mac 6 cells induced for 4 h and with the SW1353 chondrosarcoma cells induced for 18 h. However, when these changes in gene expression were quantitated the comparative values were not always alike nor close to values observed with the traditional methods of dot blot and Northern analysis, which between themselves show variability as well (*Table 1*). For example, while estimated increases in TNFα in Mono Mac 6 cells were quite similar with different techniques giving increases with Synteni arrays of 10-

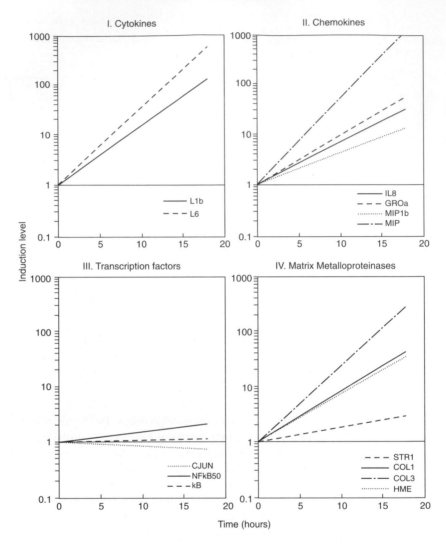

Figure 5. Gene expression levels in SW1353 cells uninduced and induced with IL-1β and TNF for 18 h obtained as fluorescence intensity using the Affymetrix array and presented as fold increase for the genes contained in the Synteni microarray in *Figure 1*.

fold, with Affymetrix chips 12-fold, with dot blots 15-fold, and Northern blots 16-fold, the absolute values for IL-1β gene activity showed differences so that with Synteni the increase was 10-fold, Affymetrix 50-fold, and dot blots 100-fold, or between dot blots and Northern blots for human metalloelastase (HME) 120- and 28-fold respectively. Details for a few other genes are listed in *Table 1*. The many inconsistencies in the quantitative differences could be

Table 1. Gene expression monitoring with microarrays and filter blots

Cell type	Induction	Gene	Level of gene induction[a]			
			Synteni	Affymetrix	Dot blots	Northerns
MM6	4 h	TNFα	10	12	15	16
		IL-1β	10	50	100	n.d.
		IL-3	6	5	15	16
		MIP1α	5	100	50	n.d.
		IκB	2	4	n.d.	n.d.
SW1353	18 h	IL-1β	6	100	n.d.	60
		IL-6	10	500	350	n.d.
		HME	40	40	120	28
		Col-3	15	300	400	n.d.

[a] Induced expression levels of the indicated genes in the 4 h treated LPS/PMA-treated MM6 cells or IL-1β plus TNF-induced SW1353 cells, relative to their basal expression levels at time zero, respectively. The increase in expression levels of the indicated genes was determined by different techniques, including Synteni microarrays, Affymetrix gene chips, dot blots, and/or Northern blots analysis. n.d. indicates not done.

accounted for by several parameters such as background levels, exposure times for autoradiography, the strength of the signal, and inevitably the linearity of the scale for each of these measures. At the levels of high and low signal intensities the proportionality between concentration of mRNA versus signal intensity is also reduced to affect these measures appreciably.

Another parameter in gene expression measurements is the sensitivity of the techniques or the ability to detect levels of low abundance genes. Earlier investigations with Synteni microarrays, using the *Arabidopsis* plant genes as spiked in mRNA into samples at ratios of 1:100, 1:1000, 1:10 000, and 1:100 000 revealed that these mRNA transcripts were all recorded as present. Using similar technology mRNA levels at 1:500 000 are detected (Mark Schena, personal communication) but again whether differences in expression levels at such low abundance can be determined needs to be addressed. To examine the level of detection of low abundance genes on Affymetrix chips, three *Arabidopsis* mRNA samples with synthetic poly(A) tails were spiked into 1 μg complex samples of poly(A) at molar ratios ranging from 1:30 000 to 1:150 000 (*Figure 6*). In each case, the genes were called present over all concentrations tested. Differences in expression were not detected for concentrations below 1:100 000. A summary comparing different aspects of the two technologies is shown in *Table 2*.

Given the nature of parallel genetic analysis, disease profiles can be obtained to address the involvement of known genes or survey novel genes expressed in the disease state. For drug development animal models of disease are an important resource, particularly when human disease is difficult to interrogate. Multiple sclerosis (MS) is one such example where high quality samples

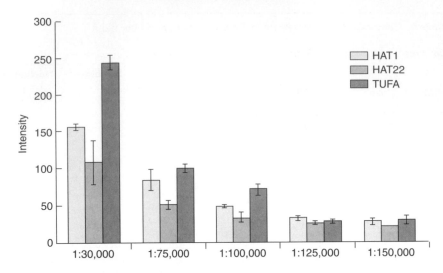

Figure 6. Detection of *Arabidopsis* mRNA spiked into 2 × purified sample mRNA. To examine the sensitivity of mRNA detection with Affymetrix chips, three different aliquots of *Arabidopsis* mRNA with synthetic poly(A) tails were spiked into 1 μg complex samples of poly(A) at molar ratios ranging from 1:30 000 to 1:150 000. The samples were processed essentially as recommended by Affymetrix. The results shown were scaled and are averages of three to five experiments. Each of the RNAs were consistently called Present over all concentration ranges, although the comparison calls between the higher dilutions did not reveal changes. Hat1, homeobox-leucine zipper 1; Hat22, homeobox-leucine zipper 22; TufA, elongation factor Tu.

of the diseased human tissue from early autopsy are difficult to obtain. Experimental autoimmune encephalomyelitis (EAE) is an extensively studied animal model of MS, in which demyelination can be induced by immunization with myelin antigens or adoptively transferred with T cells. The exact relationship between disease induced in this way and human MS is not clear, but there are many parallels that have been useful in understanding the pathogenesis of MS. A number of rodent strains and other species are susceptible to induction of EAE, and in some, the disease has a chronic progressive or relapsing-remitting course similar to MS (*Table 3*). We are currently profiling gene expression in several EAE models, along with samples of MS (manuscript in preparation). A detailed profile from the animal models and comparison with human samples should help in the selection of the most appropriate targets with which drug development could proceed.

Inherent in the process of drug development is the evaluation of toxicity and pharmacokinetics or drug metabolism. Again, parallel genetic analysis provides a look at the effects the compounds can cause by viewing the gene expression profiles of the major drug metabolizing organs such as the liver and kidney to look at the induction of genes in relevant pathways.

198

Table 2. Comparison of Affymetrix and Synteni microarrays

Aspect	Synteni GEM array	Affymetrix GeneChip
Probes	PCR products from cDNA clones.	DNA oligonucleotides.
Probe length	500–5000 bp double-stranded PCR product.	25-mers with 20–60 perfect match (PM)/mismatch (MM) probe pairs.
Solid support	Derivatized glass slide.	Derivatized glass slide.
Arraying method	Robotic spotting.	*In situ* synthesis using photolithography and light-activated coupling chemistry.
Array density	10 000 genes per array.	1600 genes per array with 64 000 features or probe groups per array (20 probe pairs per gene) 6800 genes with high density array (smaller feature size).
Starting material	Poly(A) mRNA.	Poly(A) mRNA, purified twice.
Sample preparation	Fluorescent labelling of first strand cDNA and two samples with different labels hybridized simultaneously.	Biotinylated *in vitro* transcripts (cRNA) from cDNA. Stained after hybridization with streptavidin–phycoerythrin, single sample per chip.
Hybridization	DNA:DNA.	RNA:DNA.
Scanning	Confocal laser microscope scanning for each fluorescent label.	Confocal laser microscope.
Analysis	*GEMTools* software, compares ratio of fluorescence intensities.	*GeneChip* software, compares PM and MM signal intensities across probe pairs for gene.

4. Discussion

Parallel genetic analysis is a tool that will permit comprehensive understanding of cell, tissue, and disease-specific gene expression. Furthermore, it allows the development of appropriate animal models of the disease where changes in expression profiles can be recorded with the development of the disease, novel activities evaluated, and compounds to modulate their expression considered and tested. Compound efficacy, pharmacokinetics, and toxicity are all concerted efforts in drug development. With human disease, only snap-shots of the disease are possible while little semblance of animal models to the human disease can lead to irrelevant drugs and lack of efficacy of therapeutic compounds.

Additional approaches with known genes to which therapeutic drugs have been developed can be surveyed for their involvement and activity in other diseases so that the same drug can be developed for other indications. Preparing custom chips with these genes and probing with tissues from different diseases can uncover such a role. Similarly chips containing unidentified genes from cDNA libraries of disease tissue can be prepared to discover novel genes

Table 3. Experimental autoimmune encephalomyelitis[a]

Strain	MHC restriction	Antigen	Sequence	Adoptive transfer?	Relapsing?
Mouse					
PL/J B10.PL	I-A^u	MBP Ac1-11	AcASQKRPSQRHG	T cell clone PJR-25	No
SJL	I-A^s	PLP 139-151	HSLGKWLGHPDKF	n.a.	Yes
Biozzi AB/H	I-A^{g7}	n.a.	n.a.	n.a.	Yes
C57BL/6	H-2^b	MOG 35-55	MEVGWYRSPFSR VVHLYRNGK	n.a.	Chronic
Rat					
Lewis	RT1^l	gp SCH	n.a.	T cell line	No
DA	RT1^a	gpSCH	n.a.	n.a.	Yes

[a] Animal models of multiple sclerosis. A list of some rodent strains susceptible to induction of experimental autoimmune encephalomyelitis (EAE) is shown. Clinically the animals develop an ascending hind–limb paralysis, and a transient or a relapsing-remitting course. Microscopy shows perivascular mononuclear cell infiltrates within the central nervous system. The table shows major histocompatibility complex (MHC) restriction and the antigen used to actively induce disease, either a peptide or guinea pig spinal cord homogenate (gpSCH). EAE may be adoptively transferred with T cell clones or lines reactive against myelin proteins.

and their involvement in the normal and disease state. As described above, using MS as an example, many animal models of the disease have been proposed. The question is which animal model is most related to the human disease and therefore is the most appropriate for disease evaluation, drug development, and efficacy. These animal models and the human disease can be profiled with the chip technology using both the Synteni microarrays and the Affymetrix gene chips. Both approaches are being used because they offer different advantages. cDNA libraries made from human disease tissue are a means of getting in-depth information on the genes expressed, be they known or unannotated novel transcripts. Selected clones from the library can be amplified and arrayed on the Synteni microarrays and probed with normal and diseased human tissue to check the prevalence of the genes in different samples including the normal state. Sequence information is not needed for preparing Synteni microarrays but without excluding duplicate copies of the genes, much redundancy appears on the arrays, as well as wasted space and cost. Repetitious genes can be weeded out by quick single pass sequencing, which is sufficient to mark or identify the clones. Alternatively, subtracted libraries are usually enriched in less abundant genes and these libraries can be arrayed without any further processing. Hybridization to normal and diseased tissue provides the list of transcripts expressed in the diseased tissue and sequencing any number of them furnishes further details. The major advantage of this approach is discovery of novel genes in addition to known genes expressed in the disease state. For the animal models of the disease a similar approach can be used.

High density gene chips developed by Affymetrix offer a platform for analysing known genes for their involvement in both human and animal models of disease. Currently high density chips with 6800 human or 6500 mouse genes are available. Custom chips can be designed for a particular class or function of genes at a predetermined cost. The participation of these genes in the state being interrogated is determined by hybridizing the samples prepared from the tissues of interest to the gene chips according to protocols provided by the company.

In all of these analyses, expression levels of high and medium abundance genes is not difficult to observe. This abundance refers to gene frequency of 1:10000 to 1:50000, and even 1:75000 in the total mRNA. Below these levels the signal-to-noise ratio becomes critical. Signal levels have been measured from spiked-in controls at 1:100000 but the signal intensity versus transcript levels becomes non-linear below this concentration and changes are not adequately recorded. This range of transcript abundance corresponds to about one to five copies per cell. A similar relationship is apparent with high abundance messages when the transcript abundance loses its linear relationship with signal intensity and is not reflected by the intensity, the latter becoming dampened. Overall, with both the Synteni and Affymetrix techniques, there is a tendency to observe a sigmoidal plot between hybridization intensity and transcript abundance. The linearity of the response is maintained over a finite dilution normally only over three orders of magnitude of mRNA concentration while at the low and high abundance levels the relationship does not stay linear. The quantitation parameters fall within the same range for both Affymetrix and Synteni, so that the limiting feature of the two technologies is the decreased sensitivity in detecting low abundance transcripts. As mentioned earlier for a comparison of expression levels between two samples, the Synteni dual fluorescent label incorporated into two samples hybridized to the same microarray offers a powerful relative comparison between the two samples. It is the comparison between one microarray and another that is challenging. With the gene chips, algorithms have been developed that make the chip-to-chip comparison quite practical and dependable but only if the signal levels are above the 1:100000 abundance range. It is the low abundance genes that are demanding and difficult to detect and evaluate.

Clearly these technologies provide a quantum leap in our ability to assess the actions of genes. However, their critical role in the biological process or the sequence of events leading to their action in concert with hundreds of other genes with vastly different gene products becomes a challenge for the post-genomics era.

Acknowledgements

We would like to thank Andrew Chai and David Lin for their initiative and efforts in developing tools that made it possible to start this work.

References

1. Pease, A. C., Solas, D., Sullivan, E. J., Cronin, M. T., Holmes, C. P., and Foder, S. P. A. (1994). *Proc. Natl. Acad. Sci. USA*, **91**, 5022.
2. Schena, M., Shalon, D., Davis, R. W., and Brown, P. O. (1995). *Science*, **270**, 467.
3. Velculescu, V. E., Zhang, L., Vogelstein, B., and Kinzler, K. W. (1995). *Science*, **240**, 484.
4. Shalon, D., Smith, S., and Brown, P. O. (1996). *Genome Res.*, **6**, 639.
5. Schena, M., Shalon, D., Heller, R., Chai, A., Brown, P. O., and Davis, R. W. (1996). *Proc. Natl. Acad. Sci. USA*, **93**, 10614.
6. Lockhart, D. J., Dong, H., Byrne, M. C., Maximillian, T. F., Gallo, M. V., Chee, M. S., *et al.* (1996). *Nature Biotechnol.*, **14**, 1675.
7. Heller, R. A., Schena, M., Chai, A., Shalon, D., Bedilion, T., Gilmore, J., *et al.* (1997). *Proc. Natl. Acad. Sci. USA*, **94**, 2150.
8. Schena, M., Heller, R. A., Theriatt, T. P., Konrad, K., Lachenmeier, E., and Davis, R. W. (1998). *Trends Biotechnol.*, **16**, 301.
9. Wodicka, L., Dong, H., Mittmann, M., Ho, M.-H., and Lockhart, D. J. (1997). *Nature Biotechnol.*, **15**, 1359.
10. Shalon, D. Synteni, 6519 Dumbarton Circle, Fremont, CA 94555, Ph. 510-739-2100, Fax 510-739-2200. http://www.synteni.com
11. Affymetrix, 3380 Central Expressway, Santa Clara, CA 95051, USA.
12. Sambrook, J., Fritsch, E. F., and Maniatis, T. (ed.) (1989). In *Molecular cloning: a laboratory manual*, **3**, p. E5. Cold Spring Harbor Laboratory Press, NY.

List of suppliers

Advanced Biotechnologies Ltd., Unit B1, Longmead Business Centre, Blenheim Road, Epson, Surrey KT19 9QQ, UK.

Amersham

Amersham International plc., Lincoln Place, Green End, Aylesbury, Buckinghamshire HP20 2TP, UK.

Amersham Corporation, 2636 South Clearbrook Drive, Arlington Heights, IL 60005, USA.

Anderman

Anderman and Co. Ltd., 145 London Road, Kingston-Upon-Thames, Surrey KT17 7NH, UK.

APG, Inc., 540 W Sahara Avenue 232, Las Vegas, NV 89102, USA.

Arcturus Engineering, Inc., 1220 Terra Bella Avenue, Mountain View, CA 94043, USA.

Beckman Instruments

Beckman Instruments UK Ltd., Progress Road, Sands Industrial Estate, High Wycombe, Buckinghamshire HP12 4JL, UK.

Beckman Instruments Inc., PO Box 3100, 2500 Harbor Boulevard, Fullerton, CA 92634, USA.

Becton Dickinson

Becton Dickinson and Co., Between Towns Road, Cowley, Oxford OX4 3LY, UK.

Becton Dickinson and Co., 2 Bridgewater Lane, Lincoln Park, NJ 07035, USA.

Bio

Bio 101 Inc., c/o Stratech Scientific Ltd., 61–63 Dudley Street, Luton, Bedfordshire LU2 0IIP, UK.

Bio 101 Inc., PO Box 2284, La Jolla, CA 92038-2284, USA.

BioDiscovery, Inc., 11150 W. Olympic Blvd, Ste 805E, Los Angeles, CA 90064, USA.

Biogenex, 4600 Norris Canyon Road, San Ramon, CA 94583, USA.

Bio-Rad Laboratories

Bio-Rad Laboratories Ltd., Bio-Rad House, Maylands Avenue, Hemel Hempstead HP2 7TD, UK.

Bio-Rad Laboratories, Division Headquarters, 3300 Regatta Boulevard, Richmond, CA 94804, USA.

Boehringer Mannheim

Boehringer Mannheim UK (Diagnostics and Biochemicals) Ltd., Bell Lane, Lewes, East Sussex BN17 1LG, UK.

Boehringer Mannheim Corporation, Biochemical Products, 9115 Hague Road, PO Box 504, Indianopolis, IN 46250–0414, USA.

Boehringer Mannheim Biochemica, GmbH, Sandhofer Str. 116, Postfach 310120 D-6800 Ma 31, Germany.

British Drug Houses (BDH) Ltd., Poole, Dorset, UK.

CEL Associates, PO Box 721854, Houston, TX 77272-1854, USA.

Cruachem

Cruachem Ltd., Todd Campus, West of Scotland Science Park, Acre Road, Glasgow G20 0UA, UK.

Cruachem, Inc., 45150 Business Court, Suite 550, Dulles, VA 20166, USA.

Difco Laboratories

Difco Laboratories Ltd., PO Box 14B, Central Avenue, West Molesey, Surrey KT8 2SE, UK.

Difco Laboratories, PO Box 331058, Detroit, MI 48232–7058, USA.

Du Pont

Dupont (UK) Ltd. (Industrial Products Division), Wedgwood Way, Stevenage, Hertfordshire SG1 4Q, UK.

Du Pont Co. (Biotechnology Systems Division), PO Box 80024, Wilmington, DE 19880–002, USA.

European Collection of Animal Cell Culture, Division of Biologics, PHLS Centre for Applied Microbiology and Research, Porton Down, Salisbury, Wiltshire SP4 0JG, UK.

Falcon (Falcon is a registered trademark of Becton Dickinson and Co.)

Fisher Scientific Co., 711 Forbest Avenue, Pittsburgh, PA 15219–4785, USA.

Flow Laboratories, Woodcock Hill, Harefield Road, Rickmansworth, Hertfordshire WD3 1PQ, UK.

Fluka

Fluka-Chemie AG, CH-9470, Buchs, Switzerland.

Fluka Chemicals Ltd., The Old Brickyard, New Road, Gillingham, Dorset SP8 4JL, UK.

GSI Lumonics, Imaging Products Group, 500 Arsenal Street, Watertown, MA 02172, USA.

GenHunter Corporation, 624 Grassmere Park Drive, Suite 17, Nashville, TN 37211, USA.

Gibco BRL

Gibco BRL (Life Technologies Ltd.), Trident House, Renfrew Road, Paisley PA3 4EF, UK.

Gibco BRL (Life Technologies Inc.), 3175 Staler Road, Grand Island, NY 14072–0068, USA.

Glen Research

Glen Research, 22825 Davis Drive, Sterling, VA 20164, USA.

Glen Research, c/o Cambio, 34 Newnham Road, Cambridge CB3 9EY, UK.

Arnold R. Horwell, 73 Maygrove Road, West Hampstead, London NW6 2BP, UK.

Hybaid

Hybaid Ltd., 111–113 Waldegrave Road, Teddington, Middlesex TW11 8LL, UK.

Hybaid, National Labnet Corporation, PO Box 841, Woodbridge, NJ 07095, USA.

HyClone Laboratories, 1725 South HyClone Road, Logan, UT 84321, USA.

International Biotechnologies Inc., 25 Science Park, New Haven, Connecticut 06535, USA.

Invitrogen Corporation

Invitrogen Corporation, 3985 B Sorrenton Valley Building, San Diego, CA 92121, USA.

Invitrogen Corporation, c/o British Biotechnology Products Ltd., 4–10 The Quadrant, Barton Lane, Abingdon, Oxon OX14 3YS, UK.

Kodak: Eastman Fine Chemicals, 343 State Street, Rochester, NY, USA.

Life Technologies Inc., 8451 Helgerman Court, Gaithersburg, MN 20877, USA.

McBain Instruments (Leica Brand), 9601 Variel Avenue, Chatsworth, CA 91311, USA.

Merck

Merck Industries Inc., 5 Skyline Drive, Nawthorne, NY 10532, USA.

Merck, Frankfurter Strasse, 250, Postfach 4119, D-64293, Germany.

Miles Inc., Diagnostic Division, Elkhart, IN 46515, USA.

Millipore

Millipore (UK) Ltd., The Boulevard, Blackmoor Lane, Watford, Hertfordshire WD1 8YW, UK.

Millipore Corp./Biosearch, PO Box 255, 80 Ashby Road, Bedford, MA 01730, USA.

Molecular Probes, 4849 Pitchford Ave, Box 22010, Eugene, OR 97402, USA.

New England Biolabs (NBL)

New England Biolabs (NBL), 32 Tozer Road, Beverley, MA 01915–5510, USA.

New England Biolabs (NBL), c/o CP Labs Ltd., PO Box 22, Bishops Stortford, Hertfordshire CM23 3DH, UK.

Nikon Corporation, Fuji Building, 2–3 Marunouchi 3-chome, Chiyoda-ku, Tokyo, Japan.

Operon, 1000 Atlantic Ave, Ste 108, Alameda, CA 94501, USA.

Perkin-Elmer

Perkin-Elmer Ltd., Maxwell Road, Beaconsfield, Buckinghamshire HP9 1QA, UK.

Perkin Elmer Ltd., Post Office Lane, Beaconsfield, Buckinghamshire HP9 1QA, UK.

Perkin Elmer-Cetus (The Perkin-Elmer Corporation), 761 Main Avenue, Norwalk, CT 0689, USA.

Pharmacia Biotech Europe, Procordia EuroCentre, Rue de la Fuse-e 62, B-1130 Brussels, Belgium.

Pharmacia Biosystems

Pharmacia Biosystems Ltd. (Biotechnology Division), Davy Avenue, Knowl-hill, Milton Keynes MK5 8PH, UK.

Pharmacia LKB Biotechnology AB, Björngatan 30, S-75182 Uppsala, Sweden.

Promega

Promega Ltd., Delta House, Enterprise Road, Chilworth Research Centre, Southampton, UK.

Promega Corporation, 2800 Woods Hollow Road, Madison, WI 53711–5399, USA.

Qiagen

Qiagen Inc., c/o Hybaid, 111–113 Waldegrave Road, Teddington, Middlesex TW11 8LL, UK.

Qiagen Inc., 9259 Eton Avenue, Chatsworth, CA 91311, USA.

Schleicher and Schuell

Schleicher and Schuell Inc., Keene, NH 03431A, USA.

Schleicher and Schuell Inc., D-3354 Dassel, Germany.

Schleicher and Schuell Inc., c/o Andermann and Co. Ltd.

Shandon Scientific Ltd., Chadwick Road, Astmoor, Runcorn, Cheshire WA7 1PR, UK.

Sigma Chemical Company

Sigma Chemical Company (UK), Fancy Road, Poole, Dorset BH17 7NH, UK.

Sigma Chemical Company, 3050 Spruce Street, PO Box 14508, St. Louis, MO 63178–9916, USA.

Sorvall DuPont Company, Biotechnology Division, PO Box 80022, Wilmington, DE 19880–0022, USA.

Stratagene

Stratagene Ltd., Unit 140, Cambridge Innovation Centre, Milton Road, Cambridge CB4 4FG, UK.

Stratagene Inc., 11011 North Torrey Pines Road, La Jolla, CA 92037, USA.

Tel Test, PO Box 1421, Friendswoo, TX 77546, USA.

Telechem International, 524 E. Weddell Drive, Suite 3, Sunnyvale, CA 94089, USA.

United States Biochemical, PO Box 22400, Cleveland, OH 44122, USA.

Wellcome Reagents, Langley Court, Beckenham, Kent BR3 3BS, UK.

Index